W0081274

WHOLE-BODY SEX

Weaving together somatic psychotherapy, dance/movement therapy, and sex therapy approaches, this uniquely interdisciplinary and practical book offers guidance on how to strengthen your connection with pleasure, receptivity, and ecstasy in an embodied way.

Melissa Walker contextualizes the erotic body as being embedded in a sex-negative culture. Taking an experiential somatic approach, this book helps readers map the erotic self to establish a whole-body sexuality, becoming an important sexuality ally in a larger social movement toward erotic inclusiveness. This groundbreaking text illuminates how to shed the harmful messages that an individual has internalized about their sexuality, to learn the language of their somatic self, and begin to build a whole-body appreciation for their creative potential.

Filled with questions, guided experientials, and map-building practices that help readers learn more about themselves, this book is essential reading for sex therapists to navigate the vast map of sexuality to create true health and sexual evolution.

Melissa Walker, MA, LPC, CST, R-DMT, is a somatic sex and relationship therapist and educator with a private practice in Colorado, USA, where she lives with her partner and daughter.

'Melissa Walker's book is a delicious groundbreaker, and a profound resource for all of us. Not just about having sex, this book looks at our erotic natures as we navigate our daily lives. It includes all genders, orientations, and interests in its exploration of how we inhabit our bodies from within in order to call forth erotic experiences and expressions, both as self-affirmation and relational depth. A must read, and a must experience.'
—**Christine Caldwell**, Ph.D., BC-DMT, LPC, NCC, ACS, founder and professor emeritus of the Somatic Counseling Program at Naropa University in Boulder, CO, author of *Getting Our Bodies Back*, *Getting in Touch*, *Body and Oppression*, and *Bodyfulness*

'Rarely do I come across a sex-positive, pleasure-focused resource that is clinically relevant and effective, as well as relatable and inspiring. *Whole-Body Sex* prompts an invaluable journey for readers to know their erotic bodies, ask for what they want, and have the great sex they deserve. Thank you, Melissa, for writing a book that is as refreshing as it is necessary.'
—**Holly Richmond**, Ph.D., somatic psychologist, licensed marriage and family therapist, certified sex therapist

'*Whole-Body Sex: Somatic Sex Therapy and the Lost Language of the Erotic Body* by Melissa Walker offers a compelling and transformative narrative towards embodiment, intimacy, and discourse about desire. This meticulously constructed work gives us an enhanced set of tools and language that centers somatic sex therapy and the necessity of considering the nuances of clients' sexual selves. This book is a timely contribution to our field and required reading for all sexuality professionals and the clients they clinically serve.'
—**James C. Wadley**, Ph.D., CST, CST-S, Director of Sex Therapy Program, Council for Relationships (Philadelphia, PA), co-editor of *The Art of Sex Therapy Supervision* (Routledge)

'A brilliant and much needed integration of body and mind, perfectly designed to support people in their journey to embodied, whole, healthy and joyous sexuality … Melissa is the clear, wise and exceptional guide you need. Her book is on my very short list of the most highly recommended!'
—**Sheri Winston**, CNM, BRN, LMT, wholistic sexuality teacher, founder of The Intimate Arts Center, award-winning author of *Women's Anatomy of Arousal* and *Succulent SexCraft*

WHOLE-BODY SEX
Somatic Sex Therapy and the Lost Language of the Erotic Body

Melissa Walker, MA, LPC, CST, R-DMT

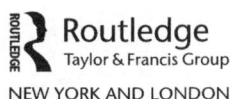
Routledge
Taylor & Francis Group
NEW YORK AND LONDON

First published 2021
by Routledge
52 Vanderbilt Avenue, New York, NY 10017

and by Routledge
2 Park Square, Milton Park, Abingdon, Oxon, OX14 4RN

Routledge is an imprint of the Taylor & Francis Group, an informa business

© 2021 Melissa Walker

The right of Melissa Walker to be identified as author of this work has
been asserted by them in accordance with sections 77 and 78 of the
Copyright, Designs and Patents Act 1988.

All rights reserved. No part of this book may be reprinted or reproduced
or utilised in any form or by any electronic, mechanical, or other means,
now known or hereafter invented, including photocopying and recording,
or in any information storage or retrieval system, without permission in
writing from the publishers.

Trademark notice: Product or corporate names may be trademarks
or registered trademarks, and are used only for identification and
explanation without intent to infringe.

Library of Congress Cataloging-in-Publication Data
Names: Walker, Melissa (Somatic sex & relationship therapist) author.
Title: Whole-body sex : somatic sex therapy and the lost language of the
    erotic body / Melissa Walker.
Description: 1 Edition. | New York : Routledge, 2021. | Includes bibliographical
    references and index.
Identifiers: LCCN 2020036066 (print) | LCCN 2020036067 (ebook) |
    ISBN 9780367276737 (hardback) | ISBN 9780367276720 (paperback) |
    ISBN 9780429297236 (ebook)
Subjects: LCSH: Sex therapy. | Psychotherapy.
Classification: LCC RC557 .W36 2021 (print) | LCC RC557 (ebook) |
    DDC 616.85/8306—dc23
LC record available at https://lccn.loc.gov/2020036066
LC ebook record available at https://lccn.loc.gov/2020036067

ISBN: 978-0-367-27673-7 (hbk)
ISBN: 978-0-367-27672-0 (pbk)
ISBN: 978-0-429-29723-6 (ebk)

DOI: 10.4324/9780429297236

To Steven and Elora: I have written this book in honor of the embodied life that we co-create every day.

CONTENTS

Acknowledgments   *x*

Introduction   **1**

1 Reclaiming the Home of Your Sexuality   **4**

Your Body, Ground Zero 5
The Somatic Impact of a Divided Sexual Self 8
The Resilient Sexual Self 10
The Embedded Nature of Sexual Self: A Map
    of Social-Ecological Impact 11
Crafting Your Own Erotic Map 14
The Journey Ahead 15

2 The Dance of Shadow and Light   **16**

Shadow Movements and Sexuality 20
Doorways to the Shadow 22
Lighting the Way 26

3 A Bridge to the Lost Language of Sexuality   **27**

A Language, Interrupted 28
A Language, Revived 31
Restoring the Mother-Tongue Language of the Body
    With Somatic Sex Therapy 31
Creating a Positive and Inclusive Space for Sexuality
    Diversity 33

The Somatic Creative Process: The Lost Language Emerges 38
Dropping Deeper Into Your Somatic Map 44
Exploring Your Embodied Presence 45
Carrying Forward Your Movement Explorations 50

4 Erotic Bodyfulness   **51**

The Tools of Refined Awareness 52
When Erotic Bodyfulness Uncovers Trauma 54
Defining Erotic 56
Enter Erotic Bodyfulness 57
The Practice 58
Erotic Bodyfulness in the Nonsexual Realm 71
A Path to Savoring the Erotic 72

5 The Whole Sexual Self   **74**

A New Paradigm of Sexual Wellness 77
Sexual Response Is So Much More Than You Think 78
The Whole-Body Sexual Response 80
Diving Deeper Into Arousal: Enjoyment and Responsibility 97
Informed and Embodied Consent 100
Integrating an Inclusive Map of Sexual Response 101

6 The Embedded Sexual Self   **103**

A Phenomenology of Embeddedness 103
Cultural Oppression of the Body 106
Embodiment, Revisited 107
Social-Sexual Ecology 108
Emerging From the Cultural Trenches 111
Mirrors to Our Beauty: The Role of Community
  in Embodied Sexuality 113

7 Erotic on the Outside: Expressing a Whole-Body
Sexuality   **115**

Body Talk 117
Dissonant Desire 119
Moving Into Erotic Expressiveness 121
The Elements of Full-Effort Erotic Expressiveness 122
From the Inside Out 138

8 Your Erotic Map: Mapping the Sexual Self   **139**

The Erotic Mapping Process 141
Applying Your Erotic Map to Your Life 161

9 The Relationship Constellation: Interweaving Erotic Maps **162**

*Four Pillars of Embodied Intimacy: Preparing to Combine
Erotic Maps 163
Combining Erotic Maps 169
Erotic Mapping for Non-monogamy and Polyamory 175
Embodied Sexuality for One Hot Minute 175
Desire Difference: When Erotic Maps Clash 176
The Erotic Map Guides Your Journey 178*

10 Refining the Erotic Body in the World **179**

*Embodying Your Erotic Revolution and Evolution 180
Crafting Your Safe and Inspiring Erotic Spaces 181
In Closing: Your Quest Begins 182*

References *184*
Index *188*

ACKNOWLEDGMENTS

Thank you to my parents, who encouraged my writing from a young age, and to my mom who always reminded me to listen to my body. Thank you to Nikki for challenging me academically and to my professors at Naropa University, who provided me with a richly embodied counseling education. A deep bow of gratitude to my expert readers, including Christine Caldwell, Ryan Kennedy, Jennifer Frank Tantia, Rae Johnson, Angie Tsiatsos Phillips, and Alicia Patterson, for their direct feedback and enthusiastic support of this book. And thank you to my writing coach, Brad Wetzler, and editors Skye Kerr, Heather Evans, and Claire Ashworth for your support and guidance during my first book-writing experience.

INTRODUCTION

My intention in writing this book is to build the bridge between the realm of somatic (body-based) psychotherapy, dance/movement therapy, and sex therapy in a way that supports you, the reader, to explore and grow your embodied erotic self. In my studies as a counselor who specializes in these therapeutic skill sets, I am continually inspired by the robust outcome of these combined therapeutic modalities. Clients who have spent years in talk therapy about their sexuality and intimacy concerns experience quick progress in their healing and new enthusiasm for their sexual potential when they switch to body-based work. Yet, a somatic foundation to sex therapy is still in its nascent stages. As evidence-based research in relational neurobiology and mindfulness practices become more prolific, an increasing number of professionals are becoming aware of the power of a somatic-based sex and intimacy therapy to catalyze fundamental and lasting transformation in their clients.

In answer to this growing wave of embodied sexual awareness, this book guides you through the integrative model of somatic sex therapy that I have named *Somatic-Concentric Sex Therapy*. I have crafted this model over the last 12 years with the helpful feedback of my colleagues, mentors, students, mentees, and clients. Somatic-Concentric Sex Therapy (S-CST) is a model that positions the body as the center axis and ally of your sexuality as the layers of the natural and sociocultural environment surround you in a dance of reciprocal impact. This model is meant to be a supportive scaffolding, appreciating your diverse experience and expression of sexuality, as you are guided to reclaim and relink the foundation of the erotic body from the ground up.

The body, or somatic self, is acknowledged to be both the location of the work to be done as well as your greatest resource. Through the somatic

DOI: 10.4324/9780429297236-1

language of the body, we identify the resilience, challenge, and shadow aspects of your sexuality. In order to navigate this wealth of information, you will learn how to harness breath, movement, and visualization.

Somatic-Concentric Sex Therapy represents a call to action with accessible tools to make real change possible. This call to action is based on the belief that the healing and evolution of sexuality must happen in a whole-body way in order to catalyze the kind of personal and social change necessary to end the cycles of shaming, violence, and injustice. When honored and cultivated, sexuality is a life-giving force that compels us to create, to love, and to evolve.

Because both theory and direct experience are integral to any somatic work, each chapter presents questions, guided experientials, and map-building practices for you to learn more about yourself. I encourage you to keep a journal to record your own experience and transformational journey.

The chapters of this book follow the concentric progression of my model. Chapters 1–3 begin by focusing on the center of the circles, the lived experience of being in a body. These chapters include understanding the body as light and shadow and an unearthing of the mother-tongue language of the body. Chapters 4 and 5 describe the erotic bodyfulness practice and a somatic perspective on whole-person sexual responsiveness to better support you to interface with your sociocultural context and intimate relationships. From there, Chapter 6 looks at the realm of the ever-present sociocultural environment, the impact of being in a body in society, and the deep fractures on the somatic self created by a culture still learning (and still struggling) to be an ally to sexuality. Chapters 7–9 encompass the realm of outward expression and of relationships. You will learn about the expressive, nonverbal language of the body, how to understand your movement qualities as an external representation of your internal erotic map, and how to combine your erotic map with an intimate partner.

As you begin your journey through the concentric circles of your sexuality, please keep in mind the following things: sexuality is the most intimate and least supported aspect of each of us. To do the hard and inspiring work of reclaiming sexuality, we must proceed with the value of consensual sex. Sex without consent (sexual assault, coercive sex) creates a traumatic wound and keeps sexuality buried in the shadow realm where wounds and protective body armor remain unconscious, undeveloped, and draining to our life force and the health of our relationships. It also demolishes the human right of body autonomy—the right to feel safe in your body and empowered in your decisions for yourself. Whether communicated verbally or nonverbally (or both), sexual consent lays the ground for greater access to pleasure and connection with the self or a lover, creates the conditions to unravel sexual shame and wounding, and gives access to the full-body "yes" of joyful intimacy.

Throughout the chapters, I refer to arousal anatomy as an integral part of the somatic explorations. Your arousal anatomy consists of the areas of the body that give you access to erotic pleasure. For many, this includes the genitals: the vulva, clitoris, urethral sponge, vaginal canal, penis, testicles, rectum, prostate and surrounding areas. The genitals are full of erectile tissue and an elegant network of sensitive nerve-filled tissue. Your genitals are truly unique to you. The arousal anatomy also includes sensitive areas of the body like the small of the back, inside of the elbow, lips, neck, ears, and so on. For those of you with physical differences or injury (such as spinal cord injuries), the arousal anatomy and access to orgasm can be rewired to other, sometimes surprising areas of the body.

For the purposes of this book, specific diagrams of arousal anatomy will not be presented in order to emphasize learning from the inside out—experiencing your arousal anatomy through the sensations you feel, the physical contact you make, and the breath and movement that you express. There are excellent guides to the physiological specifics of arousal anatomy in the sex education sphere and I recommend that you seek them out and explore the diagrams through both visual senses as well as with your self-somatic awareness.

We must also proceed with the value of a diversity of gender identity, gender expression, sexual orientation, and relationship style. To reduce us to a binary (male or female) gender construct, to a heterosexual orientation, or to a monogamous relationship style is to omit the true nature of being in a body—biological, physiological, attraction, and personality differences are a reality and a unifying factor of humans. However you identify your gender (female, male, genderfluid, etc.), you have a home in this book. However you identify your sexual orientation (gay, straight, asexual, etc.), you are welcome here. Additionally, however you identify your relationship style (monogamous, non-monogamous, play partners, etc.), you will find yourself valued here.

In addition, any level of movement ability can engage in Somatic-Concentric Sex Therapy. Variability of body and cognitive ability is another reality and unifying aspect of humanity. Remember that the movement requirement for the experientials in this book ranges from large movements to micro-movements. A body in stillness is not actually still, so the exploration of your movement map can span a vast range of ability and comfortability.

My ultimate hope is that this offering will help you shed the harmful messages that you have internalized about your sexuality, learn the language of your somatic self, and begin to build a whole-body appreciation for your creative and pleasure potential. May you learn to love and trust your sexuality and make meaningful intimate relationships from the home of your body.

1

RECLAIMING THE HOME OF YOUR SEXUALITY

> Sex is more than our individual desires, erotic experiences, intimate connections and sexual behavior. It is the deepest expression of the power of creation.
>
> —*Sheri Winston (2010)*

Your body is magnificent. You have everything you need in this moment to be a vibrantly embodied being. Without your conscious awareness, your body knows how to separate oxygen from carbon dioxide in the bloodstream, cleansing and creating fuel for the body. Your brain has a neuroplasticity mechanism, allowing it and the nervous system to continuously restructure itself through new experiences. This means that you retain the capability to learn and change throughout your life. Through breast milk, usually the primary source of food for a baby, the body creates antibodies to protect against the contagious illnesses circulating in the environment and can change its nutritional content to give babies exactly what they need, exactly when they need it. Your body is magic—pure magic.

Your sexuality is the creative and generative energy of your body, fueling this magic and guiding you to discover and participate in the vitality of life. A multifaceted, expressive wellspring, your sexuality is a medium for accessing pleasure, for seeking union, and for catalyzing the longing that resides at your growing edge. Sexuality is a source of wonder and fascination, mobilizing the instinct to journey—to go where you have not gone before. As an inspirational, driving force, your sexuality is integral to who you are and who you may be.

DOI: 10.4324/9780429297236-2

For some of you, the knowledge that you are magnificent and magical may be your home base. But for many of you, this positive reflection may be difficult to hear because your experience of being in a body is challenging—for one reason or many. The lens that you see yourself through determines how you treat your body and how you relate to your social and natural environments. For example, when you love and trust your body, getting a massage, having your nails done, working out, or having sex is an opportunity to immerse yourself in a pleasurable experience. On the other hand, when your lens looks critically, judgmentally, or even distrustfully at your body, these same activities can become a way to attempt to change what you don't like or believe others don't like, an attempt to align with an unrealistic ideal. Through this lens, the beauty and fitness industries are used to escape your body instead of being a pathway to somatic enjoyment and overall wellness.

Regardless of the way that you see your body, the beauty of being in a body is that we are consistently oriented toward growth, change, and evolution. We can learn to work *with* this innate mechanism. My view is oriented toward ever refining the pathway to (1) **learn the language** of the body—the natural cycles and processes which hold the growth potential—and to (2) **learn to trust** the language of the body because it provides us with unparalleled wisdom and deep connection to ourselves, each other, and our environments, which makes room to (3) **learn to ignite and move** the generative energy of the body so that we may interface with the world from a place of embodied connection. This pathway is not a destination; rather, it is an innate process that we can practice and rely on to heal ourselves after times of stress, large or small. This power is the magnificent and magical quality of your somatic sexual self, or erotic self.

Your Body, Ground Zero

As sexual beings, these bodies allow us the amazing capacity to feel physical and emotional pleasure, to express inner passion to those around us, and to create life in innumerable ways. While sexuality is the source of our deepest creative potential, it is also the target of the most confining social conditioning. This paradox creates a fracturing of the erotic self—a trailing shadow tapping insistently on the shoulder. No matter who you are, your experience and expression of sexuality has been deeply impacted by your family, your community, and society. When you were a child learning about intimacy, love, and the importance of touch, you absorbed many mixed messages about your emerging sexual self directly into the physiological structure of your muscle tissues and nervous system. As you discovered your body, you may have simultaneously experienced your developing body being labeled with incorrect or silly language—genitals referred to by euphemisms as you were scolded for touching our own body in pleasurable ways. While bursting with curiosity about the world, you were exposed to stereotypes, social norms, and family values about how you *should* behave, pushing against your desire to follow the instinct to connect with what was pleasurable.

"We never talked about sex in my house," Aubrey began during our intake session. "The only thing I remember being said was when I was looking at myself in the bathtub and my grandma walked in and said, 'Don't touch yourself there!' I think I was about eight years old. I still feel bad about touching my body, like I'm a kid and I'm going to get in trouble." This and many other instances had caused Aubrey's relationship with her body to be marked with anxiety and shame.

Whether or not families intend to transfer negative messages, they leave deep impressions on the maturing sexual self. When developmental psychologists say that young people are *impressionable*, this is meant quite literally; the social nervous system develops in an experience-dependent way. Clinical psychologist Louis Cozolino says that our brains are "structured and restructured by interactions with our social and natural environments" (2006, pg. 81). Our emotional and physical responses to the interactions we experience in the relational field are directly written into the brain and physical body via brain cell connections, nerve cell activation or inhibition, and patterns of muscle tension. This relational neurobiological process impacts us deeply in our younger years, laying down patterns in the deepest recesses of our brain as we grow up about how we bond with those we love and with the significant people in our lives. When we are held, share smiles and laughter, and are encouraged to stretch our curiosity out into our environment, we encode positive reinforcement which advances growth and full-body expressiveness. However, when a parent or caregiver repeatedly responds negatively to our interest in play or physical contact, we learn that our desire for creative interaction is unwelcome. The negative reflections that we receive about our developing and pleasure-seeking body impresses on us the need to turn away from our desires or expressiveness—or to indulge in private and silent ways.

The confusion created when the silence and negative messages contradict the love and appreciation we received in other ways from our loved ones can cause a mistrust in ourselves. This mistrust solidifies into an avoidance of the feeling, sensing body. Rather than recognize that a caregiver or other important figure responded badly to our naturally developing body, we unconsciously blame ourselves for expressing a need, desire, or curiosity. This is the root of sexual shame—a culturally reinforced emotion that inhibits our expression because of the learned belief that what we desire and how we express our desire is somehow wrong. We come to believe that we exist within an unruly and troublesome vessel and, since our natural tendency is to disconnect from feeling pain and discomfort, we turn away from the sacred connection with the somatic self. Like a sharp sword slashed through our awareness, we are cut off from the ability to listen to the language of the body—decapitated from the sensations and rhythms beneath our skin that tells us what our body is feeling, what it needs, and what it wants. Psychiatrist and leading nervous system expert Stephen Porges, PhD, describes how the nervous system responds to challenges in the environment: we need to feel safe to be in proximity in relationship, which allows for touch and then deeper bonding. When we receive the message to mistrust or deny our developing impulse to experience pleasure, we do not feel safe within our own bodies and therefore *distance ourselves from ourselves*. In order to maintain important relationships, we inhibit, we hold back, parts of ourselves that are not accepted.

When we are unable to understand the language of the body, our ability to navigate the continual onslaught of social-sexual pressures is greatly diminished. These pressures tell us how to behave during courtship or sex, how to dress or gesture, and where we can look or where we cannot, based on some ideal attributed to age, gender, or other sociocultural location. The presentation of sexuality in social media and advertisements in magazines displays a culture-wide striving to remain frozen in an unrealistic ideal. Aubrey continued in her intake session to tell me about her frustrations as an adult. "In college I felt like I was supposed to want unattached sex (intercourse) but I just never felt comfortable." She shifted in her seat and fidgeted with her rings as she described her experience of college hook-up culture. "My friends and I would read the sex tips in *Cosmopolitan* and they were all about making lots of noise and having 'wall-shaking' sex. It just makes me feel sick talking about it." From a foundation of feeling uncomfortable in her body, Aubrey had a challenging time hearing about sex, let alone being able to identify or explore the kind of sex she actually wanted to have.

When we live from a fractured foundation of the sexual self, we consciously and unconsciously measure our bodies and our sexuality against an unrealistic standard, and we step further and further away from accessing and appreciating the great potential within us. This stressful climate of social-sexual pressures pushes relentlessly on our bodies and sexuality. Psychiatrist Bessel van der Kolk (1989, 2015) says that "people who have been exposed to highly stressful stimuli develop long-term potentiation of memory tracts that are reactivated at times of subsequent arousal (1989, pg. 389)." In other words, growing up in a sexually stressful social environment causes us to respond even more strongly to the sex-negative messages that we continue to receive throughout our lives. Remember all the laughter that arises when the topic of sex comes up? That is often tension being released. We are too busy trying to avoid or release the tension that new insight around our sexuality is acquired at a snail's pace. Also, when we are primarily tuned into avoiding discomfort, we are not able to access relaxation and pleasure—an environment that would be much more conducive to learning about ourselves.

The mistrust of the body, and therefore the inability to speak the language of the body, leads to adversity within the sexual self as seemingly competing needs attempt to be met. The realm of the body (sensation, rhythm, emotion, and impulse) attempts to engage with what is interesting and pleasurable while the social self attempts to express appropriately based on sociocultural norms and expectations. The sexual self ends up being at odds with the social self. The result is a relationship between the social self and the sexual self which can range from anxious avoidance to disembodied indulgence. When these two selves are at odds with each other, we leapfrog among all kinds of simplistic and unreasonable conclusions, leaving the complexity of the lived experience far behind. Over time, the social self being at odds with the needs and desires of the sexual self leads to a rigid or avoidant relationship with the erotic self—eroticism being the individual color and texture, the specific attractions and desires that motivate sexual energy to move and create. The clients who walk into my office recognize this split within them and are not satisfied to continue with this internal incongruence. Though they are successful in other areas of life, they are desperate because they cannot connect with a holistic appreciation of their intimate body; they love their partners but experience difficulty in their sexual connection; they want a committed partnership but they experience instability in their romantic relationships. My client Ezra, a white, upper middle-class conservative executive who is happily married yet had an affair; my client Aubrey, the young Latinx artist and performer mentioned previously, who "hates" her genitalia after being exposed to fear-based and performance-focused sex education; or Ramona and Mark, two busy working parents of Western European descent who shame each other for having different desires and arousal levels—having been exposed to sexually shaming messages, all these clients view their sexuality through a fractured lens. Misunderstanding and misinformation are heavy burdens that prevent the erotic self from realizing fullness of its experience and expression.

The Somatic Impact of a Divided Sexual Self

When diving into learning the language of the body, you will inevitably encounter the defense mechanisms you have developed in your body—armor that has helped withstand the suffering of an emerging sexual self under siege. This protective shield weaves itself deeply into our muscles and tissues in the form of tension, pain, numbness, overwhelming sensation, or uncomfortable fluttering, especially around the central column of the body: the jaw, throat, chest, solar plexus, belly, and pelvis. This corridor is the central structure of the body from which whole-body movement initiates. The pelvis in particular is the seat of the intense arousal sensations, creative energy and manifestations, and the axis of body integration and stability. According to holistic pelvic-care specialist Alicia Patterson, "many people, especially in today's world, chronically hold tension in their pelvic floor. Due to posture, lifestyle, injuries, lack of education, and more, most of us are holding in our pelvic floor" (2019, pg. 11).

While this body, or somatic, armor is a brilliant organizing function of the nervous system to protect us from painful experiences and memories, it also inhibits sensation and breath from flowing freely through the body. For many people, engaging with the sexual self through solo sex, partner sex, or simply being in the presence of sexual stimuli, can activate an experience of distress. Physiological distress is a whole-body dysregulation experience characterized by racing, repetitive thoughts; difficult emotions; and tight, uncomfortable, or numb body sensations. These symptoms are the nervous system's social inhibition system (SIS), which we more commonly call the fight/flight/freeze response. Suddenly, the body perceives that a threat is present and it signals our somatic armor to act in defense of our vulnerable parts. When it comes to the deeply socialized and often confusing realm of sex and intimacy, the ability to tolerate distress is challenged.

My client Aubrey found that she lost sensation in her pelvis and felt tight muscles through her torso when she would begin to engage intimately with a partner. "I want so much to connect, but I just feel tight all over and find myself distracted by the littlest things. My partner tells me that I seem stiff and uninterested, but *I am* interested—it's just that my body is not."

While once helpful and protective, persistent somatic armor in response to distress limits the experience and expression of intimacy. It narrows the capacity for vitality both in the bedroom and in everyday expressiveness. The more dense and rigid the barrier, the narrower and more contained the range of expression becomes. I see people fight with themselves over how their body functions in sex or I see them struggle to desire "appropriate" people and activities. I also see people say "fuck it" and blow past all the boundaries to seek intense sensation in the farthest reaches of the sexual spectrum just to *feel something*. The canyon between the body and the mind widens and we take greater leaps and seek more intense sensations to bridge the gap and slam ourselves back into our bodies. I also see people back up so far away from their sexuality that they lose interest in sex altogether.

But, as we wake up to our habitual body armor patterns, we have the opportunity to increase our window of distress tolerance, which is the degree to which we can process difficult emotions while also regulating or calming ourselves. An increased distress tolerance window provides us with a sense of enough safety and emotional regulation to reconnect with the language of the body and heal the split within. Fortunately, we can learn to increase our body's distress tolerance. This opens a space to learn what activated the distress, how our body responds to the distress on a sensation and emotion level, and reveals better options of how to respond to the source of stress. Reconnecting directly with the language of the body gives us the opportunity to connect with a precious distress tolerance resource: resilience.

The Resilient Sexual Self

Let me say again that your body is magnificent and magical. Our somatic architecture (Keleman, 1985) gives us the innate ability to meet challenges with creativity and rest into the euphoria that comes after the throes of sweat and tears. "The body is no dumb thing from which we struggle to free ourselves," says Jungian analyst and *cantadora* (storyteller) Clarissa Pinkola Estes. "In proper perspective, it is a rocket ship, a series of atomic cloverleafs, a tangle of neurological umbilici to other worlds and experiences" (*Women Who Run with the Wolves*, 1996, pg. 205). By learning to listen to the language of the body in real time, we can address all levels of the self: from the in-the-moment felt experience, to the larger sociocultural messages, healing what we can of the past and providing a way to better navigate the future. We harness the brilliant ability of the body to reorganize itself around new experiences and orient toward growth, greater complexity, and overall wellness. We rewrite the nervous system itself and become more sexually resilient.

Resilience—our ability to tolerate distress and recover from difficulty—is a persistent friend. Many of us who experience this split sexual self can have healthy relationships and satisfying sexual lives. It is this very resilience that this book seeks to help you harness.

The inhospitable environment that is created around our sexuality presents challenges for us to overcome—this is a necessary component to fuel our growth. Facing challenges with resilience offers us the opportunity to individuate. Individuation is a process of distinguishing ourselves from others, which is a necessary part of growing up. Just as we are compelled to leave the nest of the family and make our way in the world, our sexuality must do the same. This book is a guide on the mythological hero/heroine's journey—a journey to set out into the unknown to face and master the challenges presented to you by your family and community of origin.

Effective resilience enlists the wisdom of the whole self—the mind, the body, and the embedded social self—to enact fundamental growth in our individual lives as well as to catalyze larger social change. By observing and experiencing the deep nuance found in your body in this very moment, you can release the social biases, stereotypes, and conditioning that caused you to minimize your erotic body. Within the body you can evaluate the verbal and nonverbal messages that you receive and view your erotic stirrings through a compassionate and curious lens. When we turn to the body, the place where all experiences leave their mark, we can discover the holistic sexual self that we long for.

Whole-Body Sex presents you with the tools to learn what your body can teach you about the continual, rhythmic dance you experience in each moment and over the larger arc of your life. It can be difficult to fully grasp just how integral sexuality is to our overall vitality because we have been taught that it is only about sex and that it must remain hidden. Yet, sexuality is rich with wisdom for us about what ignites our vitality and the nature of our growing edges. Shifts in sexual interest, expression, and function offer valuable information about sexuality, your level of life stress, the quality of your relationships, and your overall wellness. Irmgard Bartenieff, a founding dance/movement therapist, said that the goal of working with the body on a somatic level was to find a "lively interplay between internal connectivity and external expressivity." The blueprint of this somatic approach offers a set of tools to listen *from* your body and participate in integrous, connected relationships.

Listed below are some questions for you to journal about before continuing with this chapter. This will personalize your journey as we visit different facets of the sexual self so that you may discover a more embodied eroticism.

- How was intimacy (verbal and physical affection) done in your family of origin?
- What messages about your sexuality, your body, and your gender did you receive from your religion, peers, teachers, and the media?
- What are your earliest memories of touch?

The Embedded Nature of Sexual Self: A Map of Social-Ecological Impact

When I visualize how a person experiences and expresses sexual energy in their specific social context, I imagine them at the center of multiple concentric circles, each layer contained within and impacted by the next. Like the body of a tree that also contains concentric rings, each layer produces an organic response to the environmental conditions in which the tree lives. Our body can also be seen as the center circle being impacted by the surrounding social and natural environment. The Somatic-Concentric Sex Therapy (S-CST) model (Figure 1.1) offers a clear map to navigate the ever-present dance between your erotic body and the sociocultural and relational location in which you find yourself.

The Center: The Somatosensory Experience of Body

At the center of the S-CST map is the somatosensory experience of being in a body, the present-moment somatic landscape that gives depth and definition to desire, repulsion, and all the complexity in between. This internal location

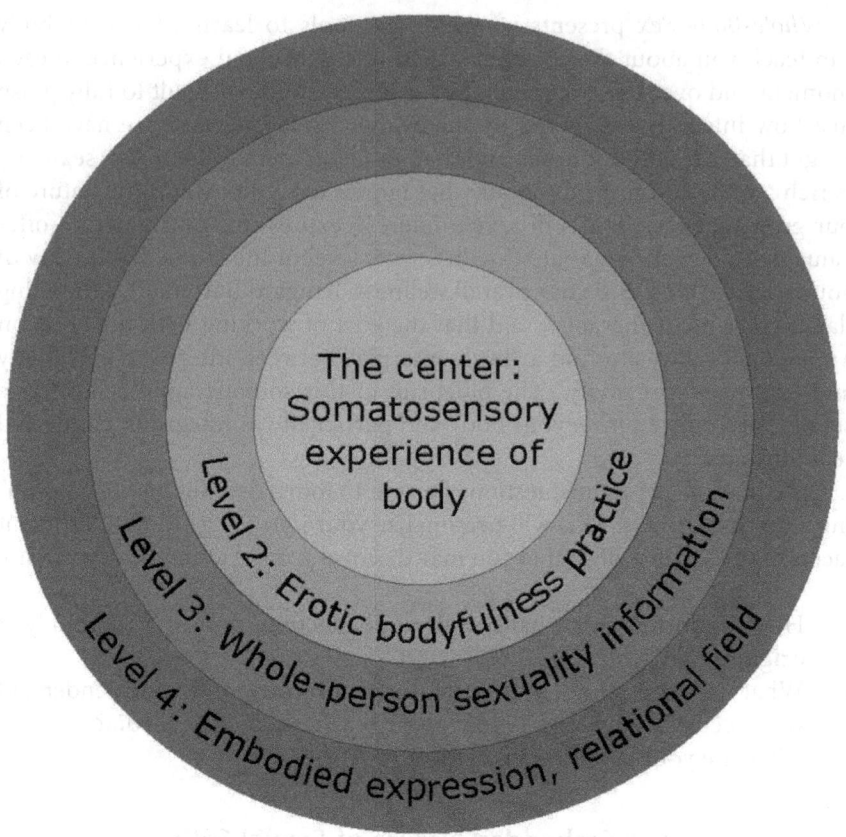

Figure 1.1 Somatic-Concentric Sex Therapy Model by Melissa Walker, MA, LPC, CST, R-DMT

of felt sense shifts and changes, sensations surging and receding, in response to the natural and social environment. The body responds to a thunderstorm during the height of summer differently than to a cold, quiet morning in January. And the body responds to the presence of a laughing, jovial lover differently than to a lover who is angry and rigidly pulling away. The more you learn your somatic landscape, the better you can understand and support your whole self.

Level 2: Erotic Bodyfulness Interface

The second ring contains erotic bodyfulness, a practice which can be refined as a way to interface between our internal sensations and the external world. This practice amplifies awareness of the somatosensory experience of the body, offering the ability to harness and modulate how we feel and respond.

With erotic bodyfulness, attention is trained to notice sensation without judgment and allow pleasure and curiosity to guide attention and body movement. Awareness becomes the active mediator between the internal experience of the body at the center and the third concentric circle, which contains information about our immediate environment. We will explore erotic bodyfulness in depth in Chapter 4.

Level 3: Whole-Person Sexuality Information

This third ring contains the sources of sexuality information that can be supportive of the whole sexual self. It is at the location of the third layer that I find myself in the therapeutic relationship as I offer my clients a more holistic perspective on their experience of sexuality. This layer of the model offers an inclusive view on the sexual response cycle, arousal, and pleasure. Working in this layer can therefore be a reparative experience, overwriting the narrow and minimizing information we previously received. When a welcoming, compassionate, and truly informative environment is created, you can begin to reframe negative messages and highlight the positive aspects of sexuality. Sexuality is fundamentally the form and expression of the generative life-force vitality of the body. This can be found in sexual attraction, arousal responsiveness, and gender embodiment. Sexuality also encompasses other ways that you embody the generative energy through creative activities and the way that you express through posture and gesture. Realizing the vastness of sexuality provides an opportunity to expand the range of how sexuality is experienced and expressed and find the health that is present in all of us, whether we identify as having sexual difficulties or not. The more we understand our sexual self with curiosity and inclusiveness, the more we can navigate intimate relationships with embodied self-assurance. We can also better understand and experience less fear when interfacing with the sexuality of others.

Level 4: Embodied Expression, Relational Field

The fourth ring is the relational space, the dimension that stands between you and those with whom you share intimacy. This is the space where we express through partner sex, affection, and manifestation of creative projects in the world. As my clients sift through the old messages they have received about their sexuality while integrating the new perspectives offered in my office or other current sources, they are invited to notice how their somatosensory experience and outward expression changes. They may find that they feel more creative, more affectionate, and more clear about their boundaries. Navigating consent becomes a skillful and co-creative process with a lover or a partner. A conscious relationship with the expression of the erotic body gives us an empowered sense of ourselves—we are no longer taken by the force of arousal or the arousal of someone else; we become more intentional in how we follow the pathway of desire.

Crafting Your Own Erotic Map

The societal map of sexuality that we receive is outdated and ill fitting. Using it is like trying to navigate through San Francisco with a map of Paris—you attempt to saunter down the Champs-Elysees only to find your body angled forward as you climb the steep grade of Lombard Street. When we have an accurate map, we can better navigate where we are going and feel more relaxed and present to what is actually going on around us. To discover your resilience and facilitate an individuation process, this book invites you to explore your personal erotic map.

An erotic map is comprised of the areas where you feel masterful, the barriers of challenge, and the wounding that may be present. The erotic map that you will be guided to create in Chapter 8 is specific to *your* relationship with erotic energy—how it has been cultivated or inhibited in your own life.

An erotic map appreciates the complex and profound nature of eroticism. The erotic is not just about pornography or sexy stories—it is a resource, the rich soil of the body in which we plant our seeds to grow. The erotic demands that we not take for granted the definitions and stereotypes we have been given but to instead turn our awareness inward and *listen*—to turn toward what awakens the senses, what excites us, and what challenges us to get creative. When we appreciate a broader and more comprehensive definition of the erotic, we make a direct impact on the negative experiences and messages. We heal and transform relationship to sexuality.

Audre Lorde, a Caribbean-American writer, feminist, and civil rights activist, wrote about harnessing the power of our erotic selves to activate our potential for change and growth—a perspective in opposition to a culture that mistrusts and works against our eroticism. To know and trust the erotic self is to shed the oppressive control of societal structures. Just as we are embedded within this culture, culture is embedded within us as sleeper agents working against us in covert ways. It is my job as a sex therapist to acquaint my clients with these covert operatives so that they can have a relationship with these shadows of society and be an integral part of unwinding their identity and purpose.

Learning to read and craft an erotic map requires the practice of erotic bodyfulness, a personal knowledge of one's arousal anatomy, the skill of embodied expressiveness, emotionally intelligent connection with one's lovers, and a safe and consensual space to think critically about and explore experientially your sexuality. The goal is not to attempt to do everything "perfectly." Instead, this is about putting in the work to develop practices that help you return to an embodied sexuality when you veer off course. The more we understand our personal erotic map, the better we are able to ask, *What am I saying YES to? What am I saying NO to? What am I in the middle of exploring?* We become responsible for our arousal and can develop deeply satisfying and consensual intimate relationships. My hope is that by the end of this book, you will be better able to articulate these questions and navigate your somatic sexual self to get the answers.

We will explore your erotic map in depth in Chapter 8.

The Journey Ahead

We are sleepwalking through our erotic life—reacting from urges and defenses instead of intentionally responding from the whole self. Eroticism as a resource is being overlooked. We are repeating the blueprint of the oppressive social-sexual system that was transmitted to us by our families and communities.

This book offers a journey for you, a journey to take your erotic self along for conversation, exploration, and discovery. This is a somatic "DIY" or "do-it-yourself" (as a client once said to me) way of seeing your sexuality. If you are still reading, my guess is that you are not content to buy the confusing, prepackaged version of sexuality that you picked up from your upbringing.

The refinement of your erotic self will be sourced from your awake and anchored relationship with your sexuality—no longer a stranger, but an integrated facet of your being. You are indeed full of wisdom and creative potential. It takes a deep rewriting—a "rewilding," says author Christiane Pelmas—to fundamentally dismantle the oppression written into our social DNA. Pelmas underscores the inherent impact of being an embedded member of society: "simply being a sexual being brings with it a myriad of traumas" (Pelmas, 2017, pg. 4). To have an intelligent relationship with your erotic self, we must approach this from both the social context and the subterranean somatic perspective. As we rewild ourselves, we must develop a living, breathing map to continually discern and navigate the treacherous terrain of hook-up culture, stereotyped media representations, adrenaline-activating internet sites, and rigid familial or religious directives on our sexual selves.

You must, and can, learn to trust yourself, to trust the wisdom living in the organicity—the growth-oriented nature—of your powerful sexuality.

2

THE DANCE OF SHADOW AND LIGHT

Grateful to be received by the coolness of the wooden floor, my body rests after a good, long 5Rhythms dance. We gather at the StarHouse in the mountains above Boulder, Colorado—mothers, sisters, daughters, lovers, grandmothers, wives—all moving through the rhythmic sequence of flowing, staccato, chaos, lyrical, and into stillness. Together, we dance this movement map created by author and theater director Gabrielle Roth, as we are led "from the inertia of sleepwalking to the ecstasy of living the spirit of the moment" (Roth, 1998, pg. 3).

After dancing through the archetypal gateways of the Maiden and the Mother, we now turn toward the magnificent fabric-draped altar of the archetype of the Queen as her many faces gaze down at us from the western corner of this mountain temple. Rights-of-passage leader and 5Rhythms teacher Melissa Michaels asks us to name the qualities of the Queen. Melissa listens with a knowing smile growing on her lips and her eyes closed as we call out who we know a Queen to be. "Magnificent," one woman calls out. "Wise," calls out another. The qualities are named more and more quickly. "Sovereign, glorious, bejeweled." And then the women begin to name the shadow qualities of the Queen. "Jealous." The StarHouse almost echoes with the word. Melissa's smile softens as she furrows her brow and slowly nods her head. "Bitter, retaliation, wicked, hollow." The quiet deepens and I can almost hear the whispers from the earth below the wooden floor. And then back and forth we name, almost in chorus, both the light and the shadow qualities of the Queen, pulling from our own lives, from fairy tales and mythology. The reverberations of the Queen's magnanimous leadership or her spiteful deeds and the ways she is revered or mistreated flow through our day-to-day relationships and responsibilities. Our voices build into a crescendo, overlapping

DOI: 10.4324/9780429297236-3

each other like waves, and Melissa Michaels raises her hand—"she is now with us in her fullness." And then the music begins as we join each other in the vertical world, hips rising above knees and feet, spine lengthening down through the sacrum and up through the crown of the head, arms carving melodic patterns around our breath. We each embody our unique experiences of the Queen as we dance through yet another 5Rhythms wave. I feel the shadows of the Crone, both dark and golden, approaching next.

Every time I join the therapeutic team over the Shakti Sisterhood workshop weekend with Melissa and her Golden Bridge team, I am struck by the ever-widening fullness of these few archetypes (there are many other archetypes and they will be explored in more depth in later chapters). Like the root system of a tree widening with each growing season, the endless complexity of these archetypes has depth in large part because of their shadow qualities; their internal obstacles and murky terrain stimulate adaptation and evolution. Each year during this weekend in the mountains, I watch women's bodies dancing, laughing, singing, and grieving as they embody the myriad of ways that light and darkness meet, shuddering and exalting at the border realm. At the same time that we women are dancing together, a men's group and a nonbinary gender group are meeting as well, trying on the light and shadow aspects of a broad map of different movement profiles in the form of archetypes and movement maps. Together, we wrestle with the edges in order to further develop our evolving somatic existence.

And, without exception, the deepest shadows that surface over this annual weekend are related to sexuality. The human potential to create is the power that is most revered . . . and the power that most tightly controlled. Through our lineages and our lived experiences, these archetypes have been abused, usurped, and minimized, as well as exacting these same abuses upon others: the sexuality of the Maiden is stolen; the sexuality of the Mother is subjugated to parenting; the sexuality of the Queen is pruned to fit tradition; and the sexuality of the Crone is invisible. Yet when it really comes down to it, all these assumptions fly in the face of the myriad of ways that sexuality is *actually* experienced at each developmental stage. But even if they are not our truest experience, these assumptions create shadows within us nonetheless as a result of the oppression of the mother-tongue language of the body.

Somatic-based sexuality work is *shadow work*. By *shadow* I mean the parts of us, our family, our cultural lineage, and our institutions that are mostly unconscious yet heavily influence how we inhabit ourselves, relate with our environment, and interact in relationship. Our shadow holds captive our personal potential, hidden and restricted aspects which were deemed unacceptable for one reason or another. The shadows that reside within the chthonic, or subterranean, depths are phenomenon like our direct experiences of marginalized or assaulted sexuality, cultural or family taboos, unresolved lineage material, institutionalized mistreatment of marginalized people, suppressed impulses and desires, creative potential that is outside accepted (and perceived) family beliefs and values, and careless destruction of the natural world that nourishes us. Whatever we have been unable to explore because of taboo, fear and discomfort, or lack of intrinsic value remains unknown to us and therefore both frightening and intriguing—thus our shadows lengthen and deepen. In *A Little Book on the Human Shadow*, Robert Bly (1988) talked about these shadows as the long bag that we drag behind us, creating a burden on our vitality and expressiveness. Carl Jung, who originated the use of the term *shadow* within psychology, said that the shadow is "the invisible saurian tail that man still drags behind him. Carefully amputated, it becomes the healing serpent of the mysteries." In short, unaddressed shadows hold us back from actualizing the fullness of our potential. But, if the "amputated" shadow is carefully worked with, as Jung (1952) says, it can hold the power to heal.

Because both the body and sex have been marginalized within us at varying levels, it is no accident that they are heavily represented in shadow territory. These creative and instinctive depths have been culturally vilified for centuries. We see this in the disconnected way that we speak about the body—we *other* our body as being separate, and often in opposition, to our mind. We cover the body with synthetic and sanitary products and modify the body to fit socialized ideals rather than listening to and speaking *from* the body with the moment-to-moment wisdom that the somatic self offers. We also see sex and the body denounced in the way that sexual education has historically been presented—like a slice of Swiss cheese, full of holes—where the topics of consent, pleasure, and healthy relationship should be. Buried in plain sight within societies, these black holes of missing and suppressed information form some of the biggest obstacles within the personal sexual shadow, pushing our most inspiring parts down to the bottom of the unconscious. These black holes within the self engulf our light.

Working with our internal shadow is to shine a light on the places where we take our histories for granted—the places around which we build strict walls to contain the unconscious material until we are ready to deal with it. Often, personal shadows are rooted in unspoken family or social system dynamics where the withholding or denial of information and experience is meant to hide a transgression or a wrongdoing. When the story is known and spoken, we can see outright shaming, demeaning, or denial as a response. When the story is not evident, the *energy* of the withholding still remains—perhaps in the form of tight muscles, numbness, or unconscious acting out by members of the family system. In my work with clients, the most dramatic growth occurs when a piece of a shadow is uncovered.

When I worked with Ryan and Maya, a white, consensually monogamous couple in their early 30s, they wanted to work on something many people in relationship struggle with: trust. I noticed in session that when Maya would travel for business, Ryan would inevitably start a fight with her before she left. The fights were about trivial things, but the expression of anger and separation was strong. Ryan said, "I feel like she just rushes out, like she's hiding something. Like she's so excited to get away from me." Maya reported feeling confused by this. She would reach out to initiate a kiss, but he would brush her off. When she returned, having missed his presence, Maya would initiate sex and afterward would experience Ryan as cold. Ryan said that when Maya wanted sex right after getting home, he found himself questioning her motives. Both believed that their relationship was otherwise in a very good place. What was going on?

I asked them both if these feelings surrounding Maya's business trips felt familiar to them. We explored the body armoring that is activated in these moments, the patterns of tension and energy in each of their somatic experience. After some exploration, Ryan was reminded of when his dad left on business trips, often marked by a fight between his parents. Ryan found out as an adult that his dad had been having affairs while he was away. Ryan had instant tears as he recalled this. Surprised, Ryan said, "Shit, I'm making the assumption that Maya is cheating."

The shadows of sexuality take root in family systems after affairs, sexual abuse, shunning of conversations around menstruation, puberty, sexual behavior among adolescents, shaming of self-pleasuring, and body types, just to name a few. These are the things you, your family, or your society could not bear to remember, acknowledge, or feel. These are also the things that you felt in your family that you only have indirect knowledge of—vague and incomplete family stories or missing portions of family timelines. Like Ryan, we do not have to directly experience something to be impacted by it. The story of a parent's affair or of a grandparent's sexual assault did not directly happen to us, but we do feel the impact of this knowledge and the impact of the rigid, protective way our parent or grandparent may hold their body when they talk about a certain period of their life.

Sexuality shadows are also rooted in racial and social dynamics—for example, the exoticization of people of color or those who are gender nonconforming. These are the roots that grow into an "othering" of the sexual self, asking us to split ourselves in two so we do not have to face the complex origins of our sexual and relational problems.

The underlying neurobiological mechanism of shadow creation is a brilliant way that our bodies protect us and help us adapt. The body has what somatic teacher and trauma specialist Staci Haines calls the "emotional immune system response" (*Healing Sex*, 2007, pg. 37). In response to overwhelmingly stressful conditions, activity increases in the amygdala, which interrupts the pathway to the prefrontal cortex—the conscious executive functioning area of the brain. In other words, we respond to the unknown or perceived threat like an ostrich putting its head in the sand: we sense that something threatening is there, but we can no longer see or identify it.

It is important to know that the shadow not only contains our darkness, it also contains our unrealized potential—our greatest gifts which we learn to suppress because we experience ourselves as "too big" or "too bright" in the relational space. This "golden shadow," when accidentally revealed, may be quickly covered over with downcast eyes, a dismissive shrugged shoulder, a cavernous hollow in the chest, and a twisting away in the upper body. Just as quickly as we expand into the space, we shrink away from the space we filled up within a relationship. We press the somatosensory experience of the body down into the shadow of the unconscious because, as Roth (1998) says, "for many of us, the body is a feared enemy whose instincts, impulses, hungers are to be conquered, tamed, trained for service, beaten into submission" (pg. 31).

Author and psychologist John P. Conger says in *The Body as Shadow*, "the body *is* shadow insofar as it contains the tragic history of how the spontaneous surging of life energy is murdered and rejected in a hundred ways until the body becomes a deadened object (pg. 85)" (Zweig & Abrams, 1991). While not all of us are fully deadened, so many of us are certainly muted in both felt experience and expression, in a narrowed repertoire of movement and emotion. As Conger says, the body itself *is* shadow, not only because of its tragic history but also because of its muscular and cellular reality. Both on and beneath our skin are a billion different processes busy at work creating, replicating, detoxing, and sending messages throughout our entire body. As a result of these busy bodies, we have many sensations, moods, and movement impulses—some we understand and trust, while others can be confusing and misleading. Our bodies *are* our unconscious selves. While these unknown, disowned, or unaware parts of us hang out in the dark of the unconscious, they can have important impact on how we view and experience sex and sexuality. We lash out at our lovers like a scorpion tail, we become sloppy in our consideration of another's body sovereignty, and the true beauty of sexuality becomes ever elusive. We are groping around in the shadows together, so afraid to bump into each other's nakedness that we pull into the midline or twist away from each other until we tire in our efforts to avoid and whiplash into each other.

Shadow Movements and Sexuality

Our minds alone cannot access these dark corners of our whole self because the literal stories are often unattainable—it's just a *feeling*, and an often overwhelming feeling at that. While some components of the shadow may appear in explicit memories, it primarily resides in the implicit self, encoded in our dreams and the somatic nervous system in the form of body memories and movement patterns. Therefore, it is the body that has everything we need to dive into these chthonic depths when we have enough skills and just enough safety to make the plunge. The body is both compass and landscape, directing us to the caverns and swamps of our shadow self to uncover the lost pieces of our life. To begin this Arthur Conan Doyle-style detective journey, we can look first to the unintentional movements of the body. Like Sherlock Holmes, we compile the clues to flesh out the whole picture. *"Never trust to general impressions, my boy,"* Holmes says, *"but concentrate yourself upon details."*

Austro-Hungarian dance artist and theorist Rudolf Laban identified the *shadow movement* that signals to the unconscious self and interrupts our social veneer, like a pebble dropped into a pond. Through shadow movements, Laban said that "inner impulses do reveal themselves . . . whether that movement is large and intended movement, or whether that movement is fleeting, small, less intentional movement that surrounds and perhaps frames the major movement" (Hackney, 2003, pg. 44). Shifts in posture, telltale hand gestures, the scrunching of the nose, or the sudden tilt of the head, these shadow movements, though small, can be detected and explored to reveal a more congruent truth. As we explore shadow movements, symbolic actions and images begin to surface. Palms momentarily facing out in front of a tight chest become a shield, a chin jutting skyward from a tight throat becomes a moment of drowning in an unfriendly sea, and a pelvis tilting back with a shrinking solar plexus is an impulse toward the protective fetal position and a desire to curl inward like an ammonite. These are not just symbolic shapes made by the body; they are lived, embodied realities.

Shadow movements also include what Paul Ekman describes as microexpressions. These are "facial expressions that occur within a fraction of a second. This involuntary emotional leakage exposes a person's true emotions" (2003). No matter how hard we consciously or unconsciously try to mask our inner selves, the body always expresses what it truly feels. But this cannot be taken at *face* value—the reasons for what is expressed are varied and cannot be assumed. When Maya would express anxiousness when Ryan would become angry before her business trips, her wide eyes and tentative touches on his arm were not an indication of her hiding something; they were a response to anticipating their habitual fight and her desire to appease him.

Learning to speak the language of the erotic body gives the shadow a clear voice about what it is and what it needs—what has been scary and unknown now has a way to communicate about itself clearly. This is a crucial step to knitting together the body and mind as well as relationships that may become fractured. Inevitably, the shadows within us are also the locations of our most valuable brilliance. When we free up the heaviness of a personal, familial, or social burden, there is more of us available to be curious, to be playful, to be loved.

Doorways to the Shadow

Luckily, when we know where to look, the doorway to your sexuality shadow can be found. And paradoxically, these doorways can present themselves to you as obstacles in the form of rigid beliefs, erotic fantasies, a feeling of revulsion, or an overreaction to an emotionally evocative situation.

Obstacles in the Erotic

One doorway to the shadow can be found in the work of late author and sex therapist Jack Morin. In his equation of a Core Erotic Theme—attraction plus an obstacle equals sexual excitement (Morin, 1996)—the shadow is a resident in the realm of the obstacle. He invites consideration of peak erotic experiences, fantasies, or dreams in your life. More than likely, your most compelling erotic fantasies include a common theme that is a cultural or familial taboo, like desiring someone else's partner whom you don't have sexual access to or a type of sexual experience that you've only heard whispered at the edges of social life. The rigid beliefs of a society that feed a taboo are a knee-jerk reaction to a deep misunderstanding and mistrust of sexuality, so wrestling with these taboos become the fodder of the obstacle aspect of eroticism.

Such complex situations are tricky to navigate and have roots in the shadow territory created by the social constructs of our culture. The challenge found in the erotic evokes feelings like anxiety, adrenaline, embarrassment, or shame, along with sexual arousal or intense interest. The student attracted to a teacher, the person having an affair, a fantasy of being dominated or dominating, or being caught self-pleasuring in a semipublic space. Morin's equation presents the complexity and the wisdom of what we find erotic. It helps us build up creative energy, tackle a challenge, and discover the release and integration on the other side.

The erotic is more than just sensation and pleasure; it is a map to show what personal and sexual challenges are the next to face to be fully embodied. This map guides us over the thresholds that we face as humans traveling from one developmental stage to another. Safely exploring the shadow to unlock erotic evolution can happen in the visualization and study of sexual fantasies.

Sexual Fantasies

Fantasies themselves are gateways into the shadow. Whether or not we consensually act out fantasies (remember: nonconsensual sexual behavior keeps sexuality in shadow realm), it is the experience of the somatic self with the symbolic elements of the fantasy that hold the gems. As we learn to speak the mother-tongue language of the body, to mindfully follow sensation and movement impulse to fuller expression, we are equipped to face these obstacles and pull the personal gems from our exploration. I often encourage my clients to really let themselves explore their fantasies during their solo sex time—to let their whole somatic landscape light up—so that they can follow the arc and evolution of their most challenging obstacles and deepest desires. As experiential sex therapist and professor Peggy Kleinplatz (2012) says, "The longer fantasies are hidden away and kept remote from conscious exploration, the more monstrous, dangerous, and taboo they seem to become" (pg. 111).

When shadow appears, the invitation is to slow down and zoom in with awareness to learn the roots of the unconscious material when it surfaces. We follow the lead of the body, awake and aware, all the way to the period of rest after erotic activation.

These fantasies can also be explored with a fully consenting partner—the key is that both parties are consensual in their agreements and aware in the moment in order to truly shine light on the shadows.

Fantasies, like dream images, reveal the unconscious conundrums that contain the fuel for your personal growth. Consider the obstacle within your most intriguing sexual fantasy or dream and ask yourself the following questions:

- Who is in the fantasy and what are their physical, personal, and social position qualities?
- Where does the fantasy take place? What are the qualities of the location?
- What is happening in the fantasy and what feels the most interesting/activating/arousing to me?
- What are the sensations and movement qualities that I experience in response to the first three questions?

Obstacles of the Non-Erotic Kind

Another doorway to the sexual shadow is found within obstacles that present themselves in nonarousing or even erotically revulsive forms. For example, I have clients who experience extreme discomfort when naked in front of their partners, find themselves turned off or even numb during certain sexual positions or forms of body contact, or dissociate (disconnect from bodily or self-awareness) when they become sexually aroused. These are examples of what sex educator Emily Nagoski (2015) calls the *brakes* in her Dual Control model of arousal.

Based on the polyvagal theory of the nervous system (Porges, 2011), Nagoski's Dual Control model identifies the sexual accelerators and brakes that work together to modulate sexual responsiveness depending on the safety and excitement of the environment. The accelerators are the things that activate the Sexual Excitation System (SES), giving the individual the green light to be turned on and sexually responsive. Accelerators can be the enjoyment you get from a massage, a certain scent, or sweet words from a lover. The other nervous system strategy, the obstacles, are the things that activate the Sexual Inhibition System (SIS), when the body tells us that we do not have the bandwidth or do not feel safe enough to be turned on and so we ready to fight, run away, or freeze until the unsafe conditions pass. You may notice your brakes activate in response to the things that feel stressful, noxious, or uncomfortable.

Your accelerators and breaks have been formed through your somatic experiences and are therefore an expression of your mother-tongue language on your somatic map. Ask yourself the following:

- What are my accelerators? Who are the people, and what are the places, activities, and things that inspire me to feel relaxed, excited, warm, tingly, aroused, and pleasurably embodied or turned on?

  - Describe the sensation of being pleasurably embodied in as great sensory detail as possible.

- What are my brakes? Who or what causes me to feel physically or emotionally drained, annoyed, frustrated, angry, or distracted and uncomfortably disembodied or turned off?

  - Describe the sensation of being turned off in as great sensory detail as possible, also noticing when sensation is undetectable or you feel distracted or disembodied.

The Shadow in Overreaction

Yet another place that the shadow reveals itself is in the situations where we feel as though we are responding with reactivity—an overwhelming emotional experience that feels too large and too intense to fit the current situation. The shadow may surface when we swat our partner's hand away from intimate touch without being able to put words to what we are saying "no" to. This is the sort of moment when we may be reacting from a place within us that was injured in the past. While past situations are long gone, and we feel we have resolved old hurts, we may still be harboring the wounds (and our somatic armor) in our shadow. The old phrase "out of sight, out of mind" may be true, but our old experiences are still very much alive in our somatic landscape. We could say that "out of sight, buried in the body" is more accurate.

You may also be reacting from a place that is detecting the shadow in your partner. Projecting assumptions onto our partner's or lover's motives and beliefs is a common, and normal, occurrence. Yet even in long-term relationships, we can misunderstand or make incorrect assumptions about our partner, no matter how well we think we know them. This is where it is important to use a mindful approach in discerning whether assumptions are true or incorrect. "They only want me for sex" or "they don't really desire me" are statements that I often hear, alerting me to the opportunity to guide my clients in somatic self-reflection. Does this feeling seem familiar from anywhere else in your life or past? What is the movement impulse that you want to follow in this moment to fight or escape the situation?

Our assumptions and projections are mirrors to our own shadow selves. In these moments, it is important for us to slow down and take notice! Do some good investigative work to discern what part of the shadow belongs to us and what part belongs to someone else—that is, a shadow that we stuffed into our bag from a parent or a partner. In the next chapters, we will explore in depth the somatic skills that can be used when your shadow shows itself.

Reclaiming the Wild Self

Like a spring bubbling up from the subterranean depths, the shadow slowly feeds the erotic self with desires, as well as obstacles to overcome, in order that we may more fully actualize our creative and interpersonal potential. These obstacles, the Gorgons and three-headed Hounds of Hades in our unconscious somatic world, are not the kind to be slayed by a warrior with a sword. These are the dark beings with tragic histories that long for fierce yet compassionate connection to reveal their gifts. We will never fully resolve our shadows—shadow is inherent in being in a body—but we can equip ourselves with the skills to make friends with them.

As we have explored, the shadow contains our greatest potential. And our wild self is often stuffed in at the very bottom. This is the unabashed and wildly creative instinctual self that socialization seeks to tame over time. The wild self is the one that dances, that closes its eyes when eating to drop into the sensuous experience of taste and texture, who unleashes its genuine sound and breath in lovemaking. The wild self is the source of euphoric creative energy that feeds intimacy and eroticism and a life of color.

When the wild self is prematurely cut off or inhibited, we enter adulthood with our very real and fundamental needs lodged in the rocky crags of the shadow realm. We forget how to play, unleash our brilliant creativity into the world, or prioritize engaging in pleasurable activities. We put our wild self away for safekeeping and instruct others to do so as well. When suppressed and unrefined, the wild self becomes reactive and destructive. We hear the fallout from this every day in the news with stories about sexual assault, out of control sexual behavior (Braun-Harvey & Vigorito, 2015), sexless marriages, and fearful or disparaging comments against marginalized erotic identities.

But the wild self, like the innate intelligence in the organization of nature, can be recovered and refined when given space to thrive. Aligning with the wholeness of ourselves, we may dispel the dark fog cast upon our psyche by the shadow. It is the love and attention that we give to our primal phenomenological body—what David Abram (1997) called the "creative, shape-shifting entity" (pg. 47), which forms itself by interfacing its own desires and drives with its environment—that makes deep and genuine intimacy possible. Finely tuning our whole-body attention to our sensations, leanings, and longings—how we *feel* as we experience the fundamental permeability and interdependence of these human bodies—opens the gateway to the wild and wise self.

Lighting the Way

Let's be clear: this is not *safe* work, but we can find the guidance and support necessary to make it not only *safer*, but breathtakingly inspiring. This is worthy work—the source of important personal, relational, and social change. The more personal work that we do to understand and integrate the parts of our personal shadow that we have access to, the more the effect can be cumulative, supporting the healing of whole societies. As the 1960s slogan says, the personal is political.

So just as my 5Rhythms community and I do during the Shakti Sisterhood weekend, together we can all explore where our family or our culture tells us not to look too deeply at these shadows. To explore these depths is to deviate from the directive by engaging vital curiosity as we walk the unbeaten path. The modern movement of intelligent sexuality, of embodied consent, and erotic social justice is a movement toward recognizing and healing our collective cultural shadow—a collective willingness to push our edges and enter the realm of discomfort because this is where our most potent growth happens. Let us, just as we do when we gather year after year in the StarHouse, explore these wild and overgrown paths together and allow our curiosity to survey the subterranean caves of our bodies and our hearts. Instead of isolating, let us come together and do what Melissa Michaels refers to as "personal somatic research." When we reacquaint ourselves with our mother tongue and therefore the ability to understand our sexual energy, we learn how to channel it with fullness and responsibility. This is erotic intelligence.

In the following chapters, we will learn how to excavate and wildcraft the erotic self. We will traverse the somatic landscape, gathering the natural beauty to be found, tasted, and cultivated. What was once in shadow will now be brought out and blessed with the warmth of sunlight.

3

A BRIDGE TO THE LOST LANGUAGE OF SEXUALITY

Where the Honey Is Stored

Beloved, we do not have to do anything to deserve you.
And yet we are always trying to prove ourselves~

asking about purpose, looking for meaning,
when all along we are swimming in the coral reefs

of your warm oceans and tilling the soil for the next season
of waving rye. This is the home we have always dreamed of~

the garden where we once saw a no trespassing sign
and believed it! The drill of the mind bores down

through layers and layers of solid rock searching
for answers. Meanwhile, a dance is wildly unfolding

just outside our seeking. Nothing to do but love them—
these bees of our thoughts, buzzing the summer flowers.

Quick! Run past the construction sites of the self
to the hive where all the honey is stored!

—Laura Weaver (2018)

Buried in plain sight, within our everyday language, a deeper language is stirring. Warm and fluttery or unsettled and grumbling, the body's words lay low until they unequivocally make themselves known. *Heartache. Gut-wrenching. Take my breath away.* And we must answer this call. Not simply body language, this is *embodied* language. "Body language" typically refers to

DOI: 10.4324/9780429297236-4

the common gestures to which we attribute meaning in broad brushstrokes: arms crossed over the chest is interpreted as defensiveness, or leaning forward in a chair with the torso signals interest. In contrast, the somatic language of the body is our original mother tongue, the visceral language of our lived experience, which exists as a subtext to every moment, pulsing in our muscles and peeking through our spoken words. Beneath the crossed arms and within the forward-leaning torso is a richly complex story begging to be heard and investigated beyond the simplistic assumptions.

The mother-tongue language of the body expresses our somatic architecture like the foundation beneath a building, forming the base as brick and mortar are overlaid with experiences and relational interactions. The body accumulates and organizes all the sensory information to help us make sense of our surroundings, weaving the collection of sounds, sensations, movements, emotions, and rhythms into an elegantly complex somatosensory form of communication. This somatic language holds our creative potential in the form of fundamental movement impulses, sensory experience, and developmental movement progression, allowing us to creatively navigate and effectively respond to the important people around us. It is this very subtext that gives us form and volume and a deep intertwining with our natural and social environments.

This somatosensory language is our foundation. Prior to speaking or understanding words, we matched sounds with our caregivers; prior to movement instruction, we learned to reach, crawl, and walk to navigate our environment through touch, sight, sound, and proprioception (how we orient our body in space). Before we understood the spoken words "I love you," we followed the impulse for connection and reached for our caregivers as we learned about love from the way they held us and fed us and shared facial expressions with us. In these early years, we move toward what is interesting because the body tells us what feels good and we are unabashedly curious and insistent on getting our needs met. You once understood the language of the body. You once knew what it was telling you. Yet over the years, we begin to question and even dismiss what our somatic mother tongue tells us. How has this fundamental way of understanding ourselves become devalued and forgotten? What happened?

A Language, Interrupted

As said by founding dance/movement therapist Mary Starks Whitehouse (1956), "we no longer know it but there was a time when movement was our language" (Pallaro, 1999, pg. 33). Despite the richly sensuous experience available in each moment, as adults we resist fully dropping into the mother-tongue language of the body in favor of rapid decision-making and productivity. Modern human cultures, especially Western cultures, are more thought-centric. As a collective, we value "mind over matter" and encourage quick, definitive thinking over slow, thoughtful consideration. We learn to simplify what we are feeling, quickly assigning explanations to emotions and sensations. Yes, the mind plays an indispensable role in the body. The mind gives us access to language articulation—words have meaning and the person-to-person exchange of language allows us to transfer important information through stories and conversation. The mind also allows us to consider different perspectives and solve complex, abstract problems. In short, the mind makes it possible for us to formulate and communicate the meaning of our lives. Yet, we cut ourselves off from the depth and creativity of this meaning when we make decisions based primarily on what the thinking brain grabs onto in the moment and dismiss the wealth of information coming from the body.

Both the quick-thinking and somatic-sensing qualities of awareness are a normal and necessary part of social living—the body and the mind working together in symphonic unity. Yet even when whole-body present-moment awareness would best serve us, we often interrupt the somatic stream of information with a snap judgment. Instead of taking in the complexity of our experience, we try to fit all our needs and desires into an image comprised of assumptions—assumptions that may or may not be true. We can, indeed, make accurate assumptions about what we are feeling and why when it is sourced from honest self-inquiry work, but, on the whole, we make far too many snap judgments. Malcolm Gladwell, author of *Blink: The Power of Thinking Without Thinking* (2005), identifies this as our storytelling problem—we human beings come up with quick explanations for the things we don't really understand. We are more likely to truncate our investigation for an easy answer and, ultimately, a partial truth.

As the somatosensory experience becomes increasingly distracting, slowing us down in our aim to keep up, the dismissal deepens into misunderstanding and mistrust. Unfortunately, as humans we often fear what we mistrust. We can develop *somatophobia*—the fear of the body and its sensations, impulses, and movements (Caldwell, 2018). Somatic psychotherapist Christine Caldwell correlates an increasingly technological and specialized society with overvaluing thoughts and ideas while minimizing the value of physical labor and general embodiment. A chasm widens between us and our in-the-moment felt sense, our fluency in the language of our bodies. Instead of placing personal value on listening to our own mother-tongue language, we outsource the task of personal meaning-making to the healers, artists, and spiritual or religious figures of society.

Why do we make snap judgments instead of investigating deeper truths? Our early interactions with the environment form the basis of how we organize our brain and nervous system and determine how we respond to a current situation. Over time, our brains increase efficiency by developing shortcuts between situations as they arise and our best response to them—the actions that we take that get the best results. Engaging in these actions over and over further deepens the pathways of these shortcuts.

The internal somatic landscape organizes itself based on experiences and our response to them. Within the nervous system, these shortcut solutions are comprised of many neurons (brain cells) whose interconnected arms (dendrites) become wrapped in a fatty tube, the myelin sheath, to speed up the messages sent by electrical impulse. These networks expedite messages along routes that become like superhighways, forming our thought and behavioral shortcuts. The shortcuts become networks spanning the breadth and depth of our nervous system, giving us the skills to socially survive and thrive. Over time and repetition, these shortcuts determine our internal physiological organization, mirroring our experiences (Kurtz, 1990). In response to day-to-day circumstances, the way the body responds through muscle tension patterns, heart rate and breath changes, body posture, and facial expression becomes more and more consistent. We develop our personal habits and overall embodied style, encompassing both our individual gifts and maladaptive reactions.

Our bodies develop shortcuts for all sorts of things like how to ride a bike, how to brush our teeth, and how to speak a language. These shortcuts are great for brushing your teeth, but what happens when we create shortcuts to resolve our emotions or deal with our sexual urges? We do not decide how to respond to the complexity of our emerging sexuality without the immediate influence of those around us.

Through family, community, religion, and other social institutions, our culture is quick to intervene and instruct us on how to respond to sexual feelings. The very nature of culture is to curate how we inhabit our bodies. Culture impacts our morals, beliefs, and how we express nonverbally as in the way we gesture and adorn ourselves, rewarding us for expressing accepted behavior and punishing us for behavior that does not fit its standards. We quickly assimilate a socially constructed sexuality, complete with a set of behavioral shortcuts so that we may better fit within our community, often at the expense of somatic self-affirmation and sexual discovery. Instead of supporting us to learn to listen to the language of the body, slowing down and supporting a grounded relationship with our bodies and creative energy, the culture presses on us to control and hide sexuality. For better or for worse, we learn to quickly resolve our feelings so we don't have to feel left behind in the pace and expectations of social life.

This becomes highly problematic to embracing an embodied sexual self as we take these shortcut behaviors and beliefs into our sex lives, performing sexual expression taught to us by a culture afraid of sex and arousal. As observed by developmental somatic psychotherapist Ruella Frank, when our interactions with others require that we inhibit or control parts of ourselves to sustain interaction, this lively creativity is replaced by habitual relational patterns which lose dynamic quality (Frank 2001). Habitual relational patterns are the collection of mental and somatic shortcuts that are played out during interactions, comprising the ways that we automatically react to the important people in our lives. When people in committed relationships say "we know each other so well," this is what they mean—they are taking for granted their habits of relating. They "know" what each other's sighs and furrowed brows mean. They "know" when to try to cheer each other up or give each other space. This gives relationship an efficiency and a sense of home. But when these familiar gestures are misinterpreted, and these habitual ways of relating are no longer satisfying or even hurtful, the reliability of the shortcuts inhibits a fresh way of relating to each other.

Relating in new ways becomes challenging when we fall back on these habits. It is as if we fall asleep in relationship, just going through the motions without considering that there may be a more vibrant way to interact with each other. Instead, the presence that we contribute to intimacy becomes limited and dulled, both in felt sense experience and awareness. We begin to dismiss our deeper longings rather than lose the people that we love and rely on. Instead of addressing the dissatisfaction in your sex life with a partner, we learn to inhibit body movement in response to pleasure, we lose awareness of our preferences or our boundaries, or we redirect our longing and expression toward other creative activities, toward other people (time with friends or other lovers). We can even channel dissatisfaction into substance use.

The chasm between the mind and the body widens as a defense mechanism to avoid the pain of personal and relational incongruence. As these defense mechanisms inhibit listening to the somatic language, they become trained against the very source of our creative vitality.

A Language, Revived

The good news is that the shortcuts that bypass the mother-tongue language are *soft-wired* in the nervous system. They are malleable! This book is a guide to unravel the habitual shortcuts and rebuild the bridge between you and your erotic body—between your mind and the real-time wealth of somatic wisdom that exists in the whole of the body as you relate with your own sexuality and with your intimate partners. The internal fortification provided by this robust and sturdy bridge between you and your somatosensory language will help you navigate the minefield of cultural and social influences and support your embodied expression of yourself in relationships. So how do we begin to resurrect such a valuable and readily available language?

Restoring the Mother-Tongue Language of the Body With Somatic Sex Therapy

On a pilgrimage back into the internal landscape of the body, we are immigrants having left the home of our bodies at a young age, now returning to our body of origin to relearn our first and most fundamental language. The story your body will tell you is of the often contentious dance between the flow of sexual energy and the prohibitive obstacles implanted from the social structures in which you are embedded. This will lead you to shed the social construction of sexuality that does not support you to find your true, moment-to-moment sexual self. Knowing your own inner terrain gives you a sense of home, of self-affirmation, of freedom from being dictated by beliefs and assumptions that do not fit the fullness of who you truly are.

In order to build the bridge, we must do two things together: first, we must create curious and compassionate space in order to hear the mother-tongue language through the onslaught of sociocultural bedlam and self-criticism. Secondly, we must learn to read and respond from this somatosensory language, utilizing it as a tool to navigate both stormy and luxurious erotic waters. This book is formed from the perspective of somatic sex therapy, which provides a robust foundation to help you become fluent in this language again. This perspective will support the original language of the body to emerge straight from the body—relieved at being uncovered and eager to tell us its stories. You will have the opportunity to unlearn any inhibitory judgments on a body level to truly see and hear your richly complex sexual self and your treasured intimate partners. Let's explore the foundational principles of this perspective.

Somatic sex therapy encourages the space for critical thinking of the sexual schemas (cognitively organized beliefs about sex and sexuality that impact our emotional, relational, and intimate lives), then guides us through the somatic map of how the schema lives in the body, and works directly with the mother-tongue language to carve a path of more expansive and integrated expression. Through the somatic creative process, these cognitive and somatic schemas are explored at the roots to heal emotional and intimate wounding and, as connection to the self is fortified, we grow our branches to find more congruent and satisfying ways of expressing our sexuality. Our habitual ways of thinking and relating body-to-body are not set in stone and throughout this book you will be offered methods for authentically inhabiting your body.

To authentically inhabit the body, somatic sex therapy facilitates a refinement of awareness of sensations, rhythms, movements, posture, and use of space to learn what the erotic body is saying about its desires and unmet needs. In later chapters, we will explore the basics of this embodied language so that you can begin to dialogue with your own somatic self. This dialogue, marked by a nonjudgmental observing attention, increases awareness of the poorly coordinated postures and movements that have internally organized us through experiences in sex- and pleasure-negative spaces.

By providing accurate information about the interrelationship between the arousal anatomy and neurobiology, somatic sex therapy provides a whole-person approach to relating with the erotic body. In later chapters, you will learn how to use self-applied touch or partner touch to explore and appreciate your arousal anatomy as well as congruently express pleasure and desire through breath and body movement.

Finally, somatic sex therapy also presents the understanding that everyone is embedded within relationships and layers of social institutions that influence relational and sexual development. This understanding becomes the jumping-off point to explore how these embedded experiences impact the flow of arousal energy through the body as well as how expression is offered or inhibited in relationship. As said by body-centered sex therapist Stella Resnick, we have a "limited relational repertoire, not only of behaviors but also of emotional expression as a result of . . . early family histories and . . . working models of relationship" (2018, pg. 40). She recommends playful and exploratory experiments to with your partner to "tease out and try out new behaviors . . . while still accessing . . . inner truth and authenticity" (pg. 40). Engaging in the somatic creative process by studying your somatic map and exploring other movement options offers an opportunity to express your erotic fullness with a sturdy vulnerability.

Let's begin by creating a context that supports awareness and inclusivity around an emerging, embodied sexuality.

Creating a Positive and Inclusive Space for Sexuality Diversity

It is no secret that learning almost anything well requires an inquisitive, challenging, and safe enough environment. A loving and interactive home provides little ones with a robust social-emotional environment to learn self-confidence, resilience, and effective relationship skills. When we enter school, our teachers and mentors do their best to provide a safe place for exploration and critical thinking about subjects like history, math, language, and music. As a result, we are poised to develop a greater sophistication of understanding and expression.

However, we are rarely provided spaces for exploration and critical thinking about sex, intimacy, pleasure, relationships, gender diversity, or consent. When we are given space to discuss sex and sexuality, it is often presented with an overt or underlying agenda that sex is intercourse and requires sexual functioning of the genitals and body, that sex is dirty or humorous, and that it is not to be done unless the partners are committed. Unfortunately, these rigid and unhelpful sexual schemas—socially constructed concepts— abound, even in many counseling and psychotherapy rooms. Luckily, there are many sex therapists, researchers, counselors, and educators who are working hard as sexuality allies to offer a different, more inclusive, and ultimately more effective paradigm of sexual well-being.

A positive and inclusive space for the exploration of sexuality requires that we address the primary and often omitted embodied erotic necessity:

pleasure. Pleasure is perhaps the first word in the mother-tongue language of the somatic body. I often see that my clients harbor the belief that their pleasure is not welcome, not okay, only okay within certain parameters, or largely absent from their sensual and sexual lives. They fear or feel anxious in their sexual body, so the last thing they will think to do is *trust* their sexual body. Sex therapist Jenni Skyler emphasizes *permission for pleasure* as an antidote to the shortcut that omits pleasure from our lives. When we begin to recognize and validate the experience of pleasure in all the places it shows up, from savoring the food that we eat to enjoying erotic encounters, the rich color of life amplifies. The erotic begins to thrive as we access, validate, or prioritize pleasure.

In order to roll out the red carpet for pleasure, we must recognize and validate the vast range of sexual desires and behaviors. Carol Rinkleib Ellison, professor and author of *Women's Sexualities* (2006), says that, after 35 years as a psychologist researching and specializing in sexual issues, the reality of sex lies in its "tremendous variability" (pg. 141). In her contribution to *New Directions in Sex Therapy* (Kleinplatz, 2012), Ellison describes sex as "creating mutual erotic pleasure in whatever form that might take" (pg. 143)—it's a sexual choreography that emphasizes transition activities (like taking a bath or stretching), effective sexual negotiation, putting structure around spontaneity, and understanding and accepting differences in sexual styles. This intimacy-based perspective is inclusive of the differences among sexual beings—each lover adds to the dance of sex in an act of co-creation, of mutual and consensual enjoyment.

Pleasure does not fit well into a paradigm that encourages sex to look and feel a certain way—this is what leads so many people to focus more on their *performance* in the sexual space rather than immersing themselves in the pleasure of the moment. To be clear, I am not talking about sexy and sensual stage performances, like in burlesque dance productions. Performance artists can absolutely be embodied, and it is a great pleasure to witness them in their craft. Instead, what I am specifically referring to is *performance-based* sex—the kind of sex that you have because you feel it is your duty or your obligation to have sex a certain way or to look a certain way while being sexual. There is a quality of measuring and weighing your body or ability against some unrealistic standard. This is the opposite of embodied sex. This is the opposite of pleasure.

Embodied sex requires shifting our focus from the judging mind into the experiencing body. In fact, being fully immersed and unselfconscious in sex is considered the most important component of a healthy sex life. Through research, clinical psychologist and sex researcher Peggy Kleinplatz, along with her team, discovered that a hyper-focus on surface symptomology by professionals and the general public is ineffective when trying to close the gap between what is deemed sexual psychopathology and what is seen as "normal" sexual functioning. For example, to expect that you should be able to orgasm at the same time as your partner, that you should be free of any discomfort or insecurity during sex, or that you should stay hard, wet, and passionate for the duration of a sexual encounter is to diminish the natural variability of the human body. Such hyper-focus on expectations reifies the fear and critical self-judgment that results when we feel we don't measure up to arbitrary standards of what is "normal" and it certainly does not resolve the deeper roots of sexual and body dissatisfaction.

At many points in all of our lives, we will deviate from the standardized model of sex. It is inevitable that we will experience desire difference with a sexual partner, illness, insecurity, a period of high stress, or other events and relationship factors that impact our emotional and physical vitality in a way that impedes sexual responsiveness and expression. Such changes invite us to embrace our unique experiences and broaden our erotic repertoire, not criticize and minimize our erotic potential. Sex therapist Marty Klein (2012) reveals to his readers and his clients the honest truth about what "normal" sex actually is—"adults have sex primarily when they're tired" (pg. 33). This is a very different picture than what we see in movies or pornography, but the truth is that normal sex (as in "average" or "common") often lacks communication, laughter, and often includes tiredness, but also unsureness, awkwardness, pain, self-criticism, and health issues (pgs. 33–34).

With all of this variability, what makes for great sex? Kleinplatz (2012) and her colleagues researched what makes for great sexual experiences and established eight components: a present, embodied, immersive experience; a sense of connection and being in synchrony with a partner; mutual respect, caring, and genuine acceptance; good communication and empathy; adventurous risk-taking; being genuine and uninhibited; being vulnerable, reveling in sensation, and surrendering to the partner; and a sense of transcendence, timelessness, and bliss (pg. 114). The respondents reported none of the performance-based criteria, like orgasming simultaneously or maintaining strong erections, as being present during their highlight moments.

If that feels like pressure, don't worry—these components are all available to you with the skill-building you will develop as we reconstruct your somatic mother tongue.

Focus

The first skill to address to create a safer, more inclusive space for sexuality is the ability to redirect your focus in a more helpful direction, shifting attention away from performative expectations and judgments. Many sexuality professionals cite focus during sex as a determining factor in whether sex is experienced as immersive and pleasurable, or performative and noxious. The goal is to have an intentional relationship with your focus—what you are paying attention to during sex—so that you can influence how, when, and where it shifts.

One of the ways to refine your focus is through mindfulness—a practice that teaches you to influence your attentional focus—which is beginning to take a front seat in the sexuality professionals' toolbox of skills that they share with their clients. Sex therapists Linda Weiner and Constance Avery-Clark describe the foundational intervention of *sensate focus* developed by Masters and Johnson as a touch-based mindfulness practice. Clients are invited to touch their partner's body from a focus of interest and open curiosity rather than a focus on any specific sexual outcome. In their book *Sensate Focus in Sex Therapy*, they say that

> *j*ust as meditation, yoga, hypnosis, guided imagery, and deep breathing training aid clients with managing stress and debilitating moods by redirecting distractions and focusing on some type of sensory information, so Sensate Focus helps clients turn their attention from disconcerting experiences onto neutral, reliable tactile sensations.
>
> (2017, pg. 14)

In their experience, sensate focus helps to calm the body and mind and creates an inquisitive and safe enough environment, optimal learning conditions to unravel the negative ideas about sex that are distracting and inhibiting.

In *Body-to-Body Intimacy*, body-centered sex therapist and author Stella Resnick describes *mindful eroticism* as a practice to support being tuned in "sensually and erotically with oneself and one's partner" which increases "the capacity to be present to the sensual delights shared together rather than be focused on one's performance" (2018, pg. 116). Mindful eroticism helps to awaken what Resnick calls the *erotoceptive* senses of the body, the awareness of sensory organs of the arousal anatomy to detect and "send sexually arousing signals directly to the pelvic region, all over the body and to the brain" (pg. 89).

Identify Familial and Social Impact

As we shift our focus to mindful eroticism, we inevitably come face-to-face with the sex-negative beliefs that we have acquired as social beings. This is the second skill to refine when creating a safer space for sexuality—the ability to identify the familial and social impact on our sexuality. Sexual diversity, gender embodiment, access to pleasure, and focus are all impacted by relationships and the communities in which we are embedded. When we switch out the microscope for a wide-angle lens, we see the individual standing in the middle of ever-widening concentric circles of social influence. It then becomes clear that we are all impacted by the social-emotional environment of our origin as well as current relationships. Boston-based psychologist and sex therapist Aline Zolbrod says that "the determinants of your sexuality are not just the explicitly sexual events in your family or personal history . . . they also include the many thematic and daily experiences you had as a child" (2009, pg. 3). She includes experiences within the family like how we were touched, whether we were given body autonomy, whether we felt loved and valued, how our gender expression was reacted to, and whether we learned about empathy along with the more overt sexual education we received. All of these influences are deeply impactful to our present moment experience of our sexuality.

Widening the lens further, we see the individual and their family surrounded by other social structures like religious or spiritual communities, civic structures, and larger cultural and national influences. This is where we locate our intersecting identities—the point we inhabit on our life map where we are impacted by multiple social structures at once. There are many people who, as a result of their intersecting identities, inhabit an erotically marginalized place in our society—"people who are at risk of being pathologized and oppressed both outside and inside the clinical setting due to their sexual identities, orientations, and practices" (Constantinides, et. al., 2019, pg. 1). As we learn to reconnect with the mother-tongue language of the body, we must consider the impact that our surrounding social structures have on our own sexual identity and experience and begin to connect with supportive relationship and community settings.

A Vast Erotic Terrain

The third skill to refine here is to cultivate an openness and curiosity around the many and diverse ways that sexuality is expressed. As we embrace the diversity of sexual experience and expression in ourselves and others, we can truly appreciate and inhabit the multifaceted nature of our sexuality. Sex educator and self-proclaimed "sex nerd" Emily Nagoski (2015) normalizes the variability of sex organ anatomy, desire, and arousal responses in her book *Come as You Are*. She encourages her readers to:

> *Treat cultural messages about sex and your body like a salad bar. Take only the things that appeal to you and ignore the rest. We'll all end up with a different collection of stuff on our plates, but that's how it's supposed to work. It goes wrong only when you try to apply what you picked as right for your sexuality to someone else's sexuality.*
>
> (pg. 185)

Sexuality is a vast and diverse terrain and it is in this realm of possibility that we can cultivate a more playful space to explore the emerging sexuality of ourselves and our partners.

Together, these skills culminate in an increase in safety and openness when exploring sexuality through normalizing the topic and variability of sex. When we cultivate a space for critical thinking, practice present-moment focus, and recognize that we are all swimming in a socially constructed sexuality that we have the power to dismantle, we take back our body autonomy and make room for a deep appreciation of our eroticism.

We have created a space to better learn, understand, and validate our own experience. Whew! What a relief. What a great tool. But this is only the beginning to the journey of feeling *at home* in your body and in your sexuality. Finding a sense of home—of comfort and belonging—is an unmistakable, visceral feeling. It requires, therefore, a visceral approach. This is where the somatic creative process takes our hand and leads us further into the subterranean caverns of the body to discover the rocks, roots, soil, and water of our mother-tongue language. A safe and inclusive space can light the way, but *how* your feet walk the path is the journey.

The Somatic Creative Process: The Lost Language Emerges

Contrary to the popular philosophy that the mind and body are separate, your body is all of you—your brain, bones, muscles, skin, nerve cells, organs, and all the sensations and thoughts within you. Your body is your movement and your stories. It is your wants, desires, and impulses. It is within the whole of the body, your somatic self, that your collective experiences land—branching over large expanses of your brain, muscles, and organs—influencing how vital life energy moves through you. This body of yours is both a play space and a battleground. Some experiences create openness and strength while others create obstructions and hardship. Above all, your body is your earthly home and it has the answers that you seek when you learn to listen and lean into the wisdom that it whispers.

In her book on *Bartenieff Fundamentals*, movement analyst Peggy Hackney (2003) describes the benefit of returning to the fundamentals of the moving, interrelating human body to heighten our awareness that "we are in a creative process at all times—creating our own embodied existence" (pg. 14). We are continually discovering and actively creating our emerging selves as, simultaneously, the world discovers us and is impacted by how we engage with it. We build on prior experiences, which have impacted our very psychology and physiology—every moment we build on the patterns laid down by prior brain growth, muscle development, immune system integrity, bone growth patterns, emotional responses and reactions, as well as belief and thought patterns.

Within the give-and-take of the relational field (interactions between the individual and significant people in their life), there is an ongoing somatic dialogue between us—my heartbeat listens to your heartbeat, my breath listens to your breath, my body movement co-creates a mirroring dance with your movement. This is what we call *entrainment*, a co-regulation where two nervous systems begin to move in synchrony with each other (Siegel, 2010). Heartbeats and breathing patterns settle into a similar cadence. This is what allows a caregiver to soothe a crying child or intimate partners to support each other. This is also how anger begets anger. Over time, this fundamental agreement between bodies, the agreement of listening and responding by moving *with* each other, forms our patterns of breathing, gesture, posture, and use of space, which further informs the relationship.

However, when we experience disruptions or rejection in our attempts to be seen or held in early relationships, these painful disconnections become increasingly integrated into the somatic and autonomic nervous system. This deepens into a poorly coordinated body structure and movement pattern which is expressed later in friendships and romantic relationships (Frank 2001). We begin to inhabit our bodies in ways that are uncomfortable, dysregulated, and retracted. We may even mistrust our sensations and impulses and try to get away from our bodies or force the body to align with unrealistic expectations. This throws us off balance as we continually attempt to "right" ourselves to stabilize and feel good in our bodies again.

Whether we are sitting in solitude, navigating a grocery store, or making love, we are engaging in series of actions to navigate our connection with our environment. Author and founder of the School of Body-Mind Centering, Bonnie Bainbridge-Cohen, articulated the unhindered somatic sequence of how we engage in our relationships and environments in a way that attempts to support our developmental needs. Her work highlights that we are in constant motion, even in stillness, as we interface with our surroundings. Bainbridge-Cohen developed a framework for this rhythm of navigation called the *satisfaction cycle*—the fundamental series of movements we make to navigate relationship with those around us. This movement sequence consists of yield, push, reach, grasp, pull, then yield once more. The cycle goes something like this: *yield* is the ability to soften and receive awareness of something interesting or pleasurable in the environment, *push* allows us to engage our muscles to *reach* toward the source of interest or pleasure, *grasp* allows active engagement with the source, and *pull* allows us to draw the source closer to us as we *yield* back again to actively rest into the feeling of pleasure to receive and enjoy.

We can move through this cycle through actual touch as well as touching with only our attention. The satisfaction cycle is quite clear in infants—they see something shiny, propel their whole body toward it as they reach, grasp, and then promptly put it in their mouth as their eyes soften into the fascinating exploration. We can complete this full cycle when we feel safe enough to mobilize ourselves to connect with the environment and receive the stimulation it has to offer. Our bodies love to experience this stimulation as it fuels discovery and solves problems. Our reward for completing the satisfaction cycle is the release of feel-good neurotransmitters like dopamine and serotonin. The cycles also induce pleasure, love, bonding, and developmental learning—a coherent sense of who we are and how we are in the world.

Though it may not be as obvious as it is in infants, this movement sequence is at the root of all adult behavior and the human sexual response as well. Yet many of these fundamental movement actions are muddied during development. When one's desires—what we reach for—is treated as negative by our witnessing cultural representative, aka caregivers, teachers, etc., movement impulses are interrupted and become truncated . . . or are recklessly unleashed. We may feel bad about what we want to reach for and thus develop problematic ways of satisfying those needs (as in compulsive sexual behaviors or substance abuse). Or perhaps we stop reaching for what we want altogether and our body protects us from the pain of this by disconnecting us from feeling. As a result, we develop *body armor* in response to these obstructive experiences.

Austrian psychoanalyst and father of somatic psychology Wilhelm Reich (1986) developed the concept of *character structure* to define the way in which one organizes and holds oneself. Body armor, which is "the sum total of typical character attitudes, which an individual develops as a blocking against his emotional excitations, resulting in rigidity of the body, lack of emotional contact, 'deadness'" (pg. 10), describes the tension that develops within the body to maintain the character structure. Like a shield or *do not enter* sign, these patterns of muscle tension weave together to form posture and movement patterns of hyper- and hypo-muscle tone within the somatic nervous system, which can look like shutting down, disconnecting emotionally or sexually, or blaming oneself or partners.

Somatic armor is developed over time and through difficult experiences that call on us to protect ourselves in relationship and in society. Like a warrior in battle, people are steeling themselves against blows through muscle tension around uncomfortable sensations. While body armor is a normal and healthy response to the boundaries and challenges of our world, it is draining energetically to maintain and it limits our range for experiencing and expressing. Body armor can become a pattern upon which further development and learning follows, causing a deepening chasm between us and ourselves.

Yet, even after many years of disconnecting from your body, it is still with you. It is still calling you home with the sensation of warmth from your hands around your teacup or the creaking bones in your feet from their first connection with the floor upon stepping out of bed. Your body is continually offering you a pathway to pleasure, unraveling discomfort with breath and movement and loving touch. As said by writer, teacher, and dreamworker

Toko-Pa Turner (2017) in her book *Belonging*, "sometimes learning to emerge from pain into pleasure is the greater work . . . pleasure as a state of being at home in your own skin, of feeling *well* where, when, and with whom you find yourself" (pg. 174). Learning is made possible because the body is malleable through the whole of your life—the nervous system can learn new responses to things that once triggered anxiety or fear, old patterns can be shifted, and muscles can be strengthened and expanded in their movement repertoire. Feeling at home is about a sense of knowing, of familiarity, of active rest. Through engagement in a *somatic creative process*, we are given the opportunity to develop somatic intelligence and practice embodied movement. We reclaim the home of our body and build the bridge of allegiance with our sexuality.

Somatic Awareness

The primary skill involved in a somatic creative process is *somatic awareness*, a specific kind of *focus* or quality of attention. In *The Power of Focusing* (1996), author and educator Ann Weiser Cornell says that "change happens in the present. The gift of the body is that it is always in the present time, always *here*. To move into the part of you that has the power to transform your life, all you need to do is to bring your awareness to your body" (pg. 9). Focusing encourages us to turn all of our attention to our body in the present moment, especially to our throat, chest, stomach, abdomen, and pelvis. Without trying to *make* anything happen, focusing encourages an openness and curiosity to what sensations are available and ready to surface. There is no need to "fix" or solve anything that surfaces. Instead, we thank the body for whatever it tells us through the language of sensation.

Engage the Process of Change

Somatic awareness is a powerful skill to better understand what is needed to engage the creative wisdom and change potential inherent in the somatic self. With this awareness, we can identify significant sensations and follow their direction to a more rewarding expression than the habitual behavior patterns that we unconsciously enact. This is the second skill of the somatic creative process.

Somatic psychotherapist Christine Caldwell offers a potent model for actively working with somatic awareness and the somatic process of change that emerges during a focusing session. In Caldwell's *Moving Cycle* model, *awareness* is followed by *owning, appreciation,* and finally *action* so that the individual may put new personal knowledge directly into practice from embodied experience. As in focusing, the *awareness* phase of the Moving Cycle is where the sensations of the body surface in our consciousness.

Owning is the process of acknowledging that the felt sensations belong to you and your body, no matter where they came from or what activated them. Because these sensations belong to you, you now have the power to impact them—a return to an internal locus of control. This leads us to *appreciation* of the job that your body is trying to do for you (protect, adapt, etc.) and feel empowered by your ability to choose a different response. At this stage, Caldwell emphasizes that "when we access inner resources and move with them we tend to feel more whole, and may begin to experience states of self-recognition, completion, and satisfaction" (2016, pg. 251). Then, it is in the *action* phase that we learn a new way to inhabit our body and apply our new learning to daily life.

Caldwell's Moving Cycle is crafted from the natural process of change inherent in our human physiology. The body knows what it needs to grow and develop—skin heals after a cut—without us necessarily having to intentionally do anything. The body knows. The body remembers. And the body tells us what we need to reach our full potential if we know how to listen. When we intentionally activate this change process with somatic awareness, new and reparative learning can occur.

The Moment-to-Moment Practice of Embodied Movement

The mother-tongue language of the body is the most robust tool in the search for embodiment. The third skill of the somatic creative process, the practice of embodiment, is the active state of alignment between internal felt sense and external expression which honors *organicity*—the tendency toward growth, change, and increasing complexity. To *embody* is to actively represent a thought, a feeling, or a way of being. In other words, instead of just speaking about what we feel, we intentionally express on the outside what is felt on the inside. Dance/movement therapy is a field of somatic psychotherapy that applies somatic awareness with the creative nature of the body to explore, integrate, and expand embodied movement potential.

As we speed up and internalize our ability to relate with the body through the Moving Cycle process, we can begin to access this realm of active embodiment. Dance/movement therapist and Authentic Movement originator Mary Starks Whitehouse referred to the embodied experience as "moving and being moved" (Pallaro, 1999, pg. 41–50). As you engage somatic awareness, you recognize a movement impulse as it arises and we follow, slowly, feeling the moment-to-moment unfolding of the action that the body wants our conscious self to follow to complete a satisfaction cycle. *Authentic Movement* is a dance/movement therapy bodyful practice that involves a "mover" following their movement impulses with eyes closed as a "witness" sits to the side observing the mover with full-body attention and nonjudgment. As we move while simultaneously witnessing our movements, we begin to realize that the body is not an object. "We are like our movements, for the movement is ourselves living: vital and experiencing or tense and restricted, spontaneous and flowing or controlled and inhibited" (pg. 35), says Whitehouse.

This moment-to-moment engagement of actively inhabiting the body with deep awareness produces an optimal state for healing a fragmented self, elegantly weaving back together our disparate parts. While using biofeedback instruments during her Authentic Movement practice, dance/movement therapist and researcher Jennifer Frank Tantia (AJDT, 2012) found that as she reported the moments of Whitehouse's *moving and being moved*, fully immersed in her movement and active imagery, her nervous system reached a state of low frequency (LF). In biofeedback, low-frequency readings are indicative of nervous system *coherence*, a balance between the sympathetic (excitation) and parasympathetic (relaxation) branches of the autonomic nervous system. When the nervous system reaches a state of coherence while you are engaged in an activity or with another person, a feeling of being in action with easefulness settles into your body. In other words, when attentively immersed in her movements, Tantia experienced the enjoyable state of full-body integration, simultaneously excited and relaxed.

When we witness our own moving body with the curious attentiveness of a friend or a lover, we can access deep healing of our sexuality. Learning to lovingly follow the impulses of the body with attention or consensual touch is an opportunity to complete that satisfaction cycle, that incomplete reach or grasp or yield, and therefore heal relationship wounds that inevitably develop from not getting some of our needs met. We can begin to fall in love with the magnificence of our somatic self. This is made possible by creating the best conditions for our nervous system to learn the skills of self-regulation and coherence—skills indicative of human resilience.

Allowing the body to learn to regulate itself is fundamental to a healing and self-loving process. As Tantia reflects in her research, "it is the act of surrendering, allowing oneself to 'be moved' by one's body" (2012, pg. 62). Attending to the body with this level of focus can be initially distressing for those unfamiliar with this level of awareness, but this is not a queue to give up! When we feel out of control, "it is unfamiliarity of a suppressed part of experience—embodied experience—that is being recognized" (pg. 62). Over time and titration (dipping into a challenge and then returning to a more comfortable place to access the state of yield or rest), what is unknown becomes more familiar, and distress tolerance and nervous system coherence becomes more common. This ability to be awake and aware of the present moment fluctuations of pain and pleasure allows us an ultimately more pleasurable experience of being in a body. When we discover these moments of alignment, there is an internal volumizing felt experience that is visible to others. A sense of home settles into our very bones when this sweet spot of our abilities successfully engages the challenges of the environment.

Dropping Deeper Into Your Somatic Map

So how do you begin to understand your somatic mother tongue, to read your sensations and movement qualities, so that you can access the deeper meaning and healing potential of your body? Embodied movement exploration aids us in strengthening the bridge between the mind and the whole self—a direction to focus a nonjudgmental attention to illuminate the somatosensory landscape.

Your somatic map is your inner landscape of sensation and rhythm combined with your outer movements, gestures, paraverbals (voice tone and pitch), and breath quality. It is the present moment accumulation of all that your body has experienced and, when you observe your somatic map over time, patterns and deeper stories emerge. You may notice as you observe others that some people take up more space than others or that some are sharp and quick in their movements while others are slow and languid. Each of these is a basic movement profile, a somatic map of external expression that mirrors an internal felt sense of being.

The process of learning the language of your somatic map begins with you taking on the perspective of a curious and kind somatic researcher. A valuable guide for your somatic research is found in embodied movement exploration, which will be facilitated throughout the rest of this book. Let's begin with the movement exploration and understanding provided by the language of the Kestenberg Movement Profile (KMP), an assessment tool and healing structure utilized by dance/movement therapists. KMP explores qualities of movement, patterns of muscle tension, pace, posture, and use of *kinesphere* (the space around a person's body).

During my master's in somatic counseling psychology program at Naropa University, my curriculum included a Body Movement and Observation class taught by my professor and mentor Ryan Kennedy, a somatic psychotherapist and Laban movement analyst. Using KMP, he assigned us the task of creating a "home base character" and a "challenge character" for a classmate after observing their movement qualities. We trained our curiosity on how they took up space and what they reported feeling with each movement. As we observed the way our partner inhabited their body and kinesphere, we assessed the rhythmic quality of their movement as their muscles contracted and released and the speed and intensity with which they transitioned between movements. We identified when their movements expressed a level of confidence and mastery and when they looked like they were unsure or defending against something. We also identified how their breath and gesture allowed them to interact with the environment and how they expanded into the space around them or shrunk more tightly into themselves. As we took turns studying each other's movement map, we looked for the commonly expressed or "home base" movements, as well as the movements that they rarely expressed or felt uncomfortable embodying—the "challenge" movements. The numerous characters emerged as a strand of seaweed in the ocean, a kickboxer in battle, or a rabbit hiding in the grass. This project helped to identify movement preferences and habits as well as ways to push the growing edges of expression and expand our movement repertoire.

Let's engage embodied movement exploration to research *your* home base and challenge characters now.

Exploring Your Embodied Presence

Let's take a look at the main aspects of your movement profile through the lens of KMP as a foundation for further movement explorations related to sexuality throughout this book. While KMP takes years of study and practice to master, there are four main areas that can serve as a jumping-off point for your personal somatic research into your erotic body: body rhythms, transitions between movement and rhythms, defensive and receptive body states, and your body response to being in relationship with the environment and to other people.

Body rhythms: Let's begin with an exploration of the rhythms that your body can create through the tension and relaxation of your muscle tissue. *Tension-flow* refers to the combinations of contractions and expansions of muscle tissue in the body. *Bound tension-flow,* associated with the sympathetic nervous system, accompanies feelings of inhibition and constraint, while *free tension-flow,* associated with the parasympathetic nervous system, refers to the "pleasant feeling in the release of movement" (Kestenberg-Amighi, Loman, & Sossin, 2018, pg. 25). Both bound and free tension-flow are forms of *animated flow,* a spectrum of high to low levels of intensity. Think about all the contraction and expansion of your muscles that allow you to run through the park—you flex to lift your leg and release to extend your leg behind. Also think of the contraction and expansion of your body when your partner calls to tell you that they can't make it to the dinner that you were both anticipating. Bound muscle tension increases in your stomach and shoulders, evoking a sense of frustration, or you experience a sudden free tension-flow as your shoulders slump. Maybe your partner often cancels exciting plans and you have begun to mute your emotional response. *Neutral flow* reflects the "numbing of emotions and thoughts" (pg. 25) that can appear as a shutdown in the body and a lack of bound- or free-flow alterations in muscle tension. Neutral flow can show up in depression or illness. It can also show up in intimacy when one feels obligated to have sex or when one has experienced trauma and the pelvis is numbed to sensation.

These forms of flow culminate in rhythmic movement strategies of alternating patterns of muscle tension in the body. Sometimes, these rhythmic strategies are *indulging*, activating more of the parasympathetic nervous system, which allows you to adapt to a situation. Other rhythmic strategies have a *fighting* quality, which activate more of the sympathetic nervous system and allow for more aggressive action and boundary setting.

While all these rhythmic movement strategies describe movement qualities characteristic of different phases of human development, we can also enlist these rhythms in the exploration of the movements of the sexual self. While activating somatic awareness, notice what are your home rhythms— rhythms that you express naturally and that feel good or comfortable. Which rhythms feel foreign or uncomfortable for you? What is the context in which you find yourself expressing the different rhythms?

Indulging tension-flow rhythms include:

- *Sucking:* A "smooth alteration between free flow and bound flow" (pg. 28) indicative of self-soothing and bonding attunement. This rhythm facilitates body-to-body attunement between infant and caregiver and, later, between lovers or intimate partners. The sucking rhythm is seen in the soothing caresses on a partner's hand or cheek or while rocking back and forth in a rocking chair. Sucking rhythms also show up in enmeshed or boundaryless relationships, soothing each other without setting boundaries to care for the self.
- *Twisting:* This rhythm encourages flow adjustments from the pelvis, twisting the body in playful teasing. The twisting rhythm is seen in a humorous outlook and flirtatious banter. It supports internal integrity through improvisation and adaptation in changing environments. It also shows up in complaining and avoiding straightforward connection.
- *Running/drifting:* The arrival of this rhythm is marked by an abundance of free tension-flow causing one to "wander aimlessly without boundaries" (pg. 41). Running/drifting shows up as meandering through a park on a warm, sunny day, allowing your senses to carry you along, unhindered, to what looks and smells and feels pleasurable. With too much running/drifting, we misplace things or appear as spacey and unfocused. We can also miss cues of sexual partners when they indicate a removal of consent or a desire for something different.
- *Swaying:* Characterized by "wave-like contractions of gradually increasing and decreasing intensity," the swaying rhythm creates "soft, flowing movements that can be seen in a languid, swaying walk" (pg. 46). Picture seaweed at the ocean floor flowing with the tide. This rhythm smooths out the sharp edges of movement, supporting nurturing behaviors and a lack of urgency. Think of unhurried lovemaking or an unselfconscious embodiment of gender expression. A prominence of the swaying rhythm can also be a going-with-the-flow and deferring to the desires and demands of lovers or partners.

- *Jumping:* The jumping rhythm is an "overflow of energy and excitement which functions in the service of externalizing . . . sexual feelings" (pg. 49). Expressed through high-intensity play, this is a gregarious and energetic rhythm which can be both fun and intrusive or disruptive.

Fighting tension-flow rhythms include:

- *Snapping/biting:* Follows the sucking rhythm and facilitates differentiation. This tapping-like rhythm alternates between bound- and free-flow muscle tension but adds a sharp transition. The biting rhythm creates boundaries and an otherness that is necessary to become independent, requesting and caring for one's own needs. It can also be seen in kink play such as flogging, where contact creates a moment of pain followed by an often pleasurable free-flow tension release.
- *Strain/release:* This rhythm is the conscious process of holding, pushing, and letting go, thereby establishing the intentional setting of boundaries and assertiveness . . . or stubbornness. Strain/release sets the stage for navigating consent, saying "yes" and saying "no" to intimate contact. Overuse of this rhythm is indicative of an inability to let go of emotional hurts or difficulty relaxing into a sensual or sexual experience.
- *Starting/stopping:* This is another rhythm characterized by sharp transitions (as in the biting rhythm), though starting/stopping is more a rhythm of coordinated control. It is indicative of a mastery of time, being able to intentionally begin and end an activity to achieve goals and participate in competitions. This rhythm appears in the disciplined beginning and ending of sexual activity or transitioning between different forms of sensory play. Starting/stopping can also feel abrupt and disruptive to a desired flow of intimacy.
- *Surging/birthing:* Gradually building to high levels of intensity followed by a perfunctory release, surging/birthing is seen in childbirth, genital orgasm, and a passionate meeting between lovers.
- *Spurting/ramming:* When the jumping rhythm becomes more sharply differentiated, an expression of focused purposefulness sets in. This rhythm is present in stronger motions of penetrative sex and high levels of arousal energy. Too much spurting/ramming rhythm can also present as a pressure to engage in sex or specific sexual activities, or pressuring to conform to a particular sexual orientation, gender expression, or relationship dynamic.

Make a note of your home rhythmic strategies as well as the rhythms that feel unfamiliar or even uncomfortable. Now let's look at how you can transition between rhythms.

Transitions between movement and rhythms: Now let's explore how you transition between movements and rhythms, how you relate to the change process provided by the existence of time and gravity. This is what KMP refers to as *tension-flow attributes*. Attributes of tension-flow are descriptors of transition qualities and adjustments between rhythms, activities, or moods. The way you transition between rhythms, moods, and activities offers you valuable information about how you respond to a change in situation. It reveals what your resilient qualities are that help you transition effectively, as well as your coping mechanisms that hinder your adaptation to different situations.

As you explore these attributes, notice what method of transition you express in sex and intimacy when you feel you are effective and which you express when you are stressed.

- *Even flow:* Maintains contact with evenly held tension levels, such as in a slow and evenly paced lovemaking rhythm or when you let your hand rest on your partner's back as you or your partner may adjust to get more comfortable.
- *Flow adjustment:* Small and subtle adjustments, as in the twisting rhythm, which allow for lightness, adaptability, and playfulness.
- *High intensity:* When combined with free flow, a high intensity attribute supports wild and unconstrained movements. When combined with bound flow, high intensity becomes a powerful restraining of expression, even immobilizing the body.
- *Low intensity:* Movement transitions that are subtle and muted. Indicative of shy or reserved movement expression.
- *Abruptness:* Swift change in intensity, as in jumping rhythm or spurting/ramming. An abrupt attribute is quick to anger, quick to calm down, and quick to say what they think without considering the impact.
- *Graduality:* Moving into different moods or activities with measured transitions. A "slow-burning fuse."

Taking in this list, consider how you move through transitions. How do you adjust to being home after work, move into intimacy with your partner, and transition between sexual activities? Do you enjoy moving quickly between things or do you like to take your time? Also consider how you transition between being in different cultural contexts. What tension-flow attributes do you express when in a group of your peers versus when you are with your family or when you travel to a different state or country?

Masterful and learning body states: There are times when you feel confident in the way you are navigating your environment and relationships. Other times, you feel uncertain because you don't know how to do something, you don't feel you can do it well, or you are protecting yourself from a challenging or dangerous part of your environment. These two scenarios are described in KMP as *pre-efforts* and *efforts*.

Pre-efforts are the sort of movements expressed when learning something new, trying something new, or when using defense mechanisms. Crucial to development and learning, pre-efforts can come across as hesitation, abruptness, intense focus, or lack of confidence. Unfortunately, sexual *pre-efforts* are often interpreted negatively by lovers. In my work with couples, we often spend time dispelling assumptions and judgments that arise in response to *pre-effort* bids for connection or sexual expression. For example, when one partner hesitates before they reach for intimate contact, the other person will question the hesitant partner's motives, their sexual prowess, or even their own attractiveness. I find that assumptions about *pre-efforts* are often incorrect. Sometimes, the hesitant partner is simply unsure how their partner will respond to their desire for intimacy because they know the partner had a long day. Other times, the hesitant partner is trying on something new and they are entering new territory by initiating sex. Perhaps someone is new to outwardly expressing their gender or sexual orientation. There are so many reasons for *pre-effort* expression that it is crucial that we slow down and practice compassion and good communication. We have the power to set ourselves and our partners up for success. When we are surrounded by a welcoming space to master skills and ways of embodying and expressing our sexuality, *pre-efforts* refine into *efforts*.

Effort expressions reveal a level of confidence in our abilities and in how we represent ourselves. This kind of effort will be explored in depth in Chapter 7.

Make a note of the moments in sex and intimacy where you feel confident and comfortable. Also make note of the moments where you feel uncertain, hesitant, or defensive of your body or your feelings.

Lastly, we can identify how the somatic self is impacted by being in relationship with another person or with the environment. This is where *shape flow* comes in: shape flow describes how your body shape changes in response to relationship.

Response to your environment and to other people: In response to warm, pleasant environments, we widen and lengthen the body to take in more sensation. In response to cold or uncomfortable environments, we shrink and hollow the body to take in less sensation. *Shape flow* describes "the movement of the body in space and the kinds of structures and shapes it creates . . . helping to understand the relationship of the mover to the self and to others" (pg. 110).

In *bipolar shape flow*, we see symmetrical expansions and contractions, encouraging balance and stability. The growing movements of bipolar shape flow, which include *widening, lengthening*, and *bulging*, "tend to create open shapes which expose the body to the environment" (pg. 113). We *grow* in body shape when we feel confident, excited, in love, and turned on. The face widens into a smile; arms spread open for a hug. Meanwhile, the shrinking movements of bipolar shape flow emerge as the body *narrows, shortens,* or *hollows,* "creat[ing] closed shapes which reduce exposure of the body to outside contact" (pg. 113). We shrink and retract into the safety of the mid-body when we are nervous, feel unwelcome, or are turned off. The chin or eyes lower and shoulders round into a hollowing shape around the chest. Notice for yourself what inspires you to *grow* in your body, opening to a sensual environment or a lover. Also notice what discourages your body from opening to the environment, demanding that you make yourself smaller and less noticeable.

In contrast to bipolar shape flow, *unipolar shape flow* describes an asymmetrical growing and shrinking that facilitates body mobility, as in moving toward or away from someone. This type of movement supports us in shaping our body in specific directions. We can widen on one side of the body to lean in for contact or we can shrink one side of the body toward the midline to avoid contact as we squeeze by a bar counter full of people. Unipolar shape flow describes how we express attraction or repulsion, reaching our cheek out for a kiss or pulling our hand away from unwanted intimate contact. Use somatic awareness to notice how it feels for you to grow your body in the direction of something pleasurable. Also notice how it feels to shrink your body away from something noxious. We will explore this in more depth in Chapter 7.

Carrying Forward Your Movement Explorations

As new ideas and experiments are presented throughout this book, I invite you to return to this section to identify what sorts of rhythms, transitions, defensive and receptive expressions, and response to your environment that your body expresses. This is a useful guide for helping to identify what the language of the body is telling you about how you embody and express the various aspects of your sexuality. It is also a useful support for the broadening of your movement options, opening a new area of your repertoire to more fully inhabit your intimate spaces. Instead of comparing yourself against what is "normal," you are invited to explore all that is present in real time and, with curiosity, follow the trail of bread crumbs to your embodied sexual self.

4

EROTIC BODYFULNESS

The simple act of reaching for a glass of water to take a drink can be a mundane or casual action of necessity, yet when I was pregnant with my daughter and then during the many months that I pumped milk for her, the coordinated series of movements involved in drinking water became a deeply intense experience. My thirst throbbed on a primal, cellular level. I found my body moving as a whole toward my jug of ice water, almost enveloping the whole thing as I drank deeply, eyes closed, feeling each molecule of water being sucked into my every cell and muscle fiber. I couldn't take in the water fast enough and my body urged me to drink more. This experience was primal, biological need, and felt sense desire merged into one master purpose: to HYDRATE. The potency of this experience was insistently sensuous as well as essentially nourishing. When my thirst was the most intense, I found myself in a flow state, focused and fully in the present moment. Before this moment, I never knew that drinking water could be so painfully, urgently pleasurable. This simple act of drinking water became an erotic moment for me, and the awareness of my body called on me to get ever closer to my phenomenological experience.

Over the years, my erotic awareness practice has been refined through many moments just like this one. As I guide clients through this practice while they relate with the cup of warm tea in their hands, the pleasure of the moment is often deliciously accessible. However, when I guide clients through this practice as they make sensual contact with their partner's hand or cheek, the complexity that arises can be challenging. Over time, these same clients uncover layer after layer of tension, every time opening more fully to sensation and connection.

When we engage intimately, we may feel the rise of pleasure—an opening and warmth in the body toward contact. A flush of heat and thickness in the

DOI: 10.4324/9780429297236-5

pelvis. Simultaneously, we may feel a tightness in the chest or jaw. We may feel numbness. The thinking mind may begin to take over and these sensations can be closely followed by thoughts of "this feels so good" right alongside "I'm not allowed to do this" or "I'm doing this wrong." When we have been exposed to negative sociocultural messages, when the internal somatic map senses that pleasure is present, it constricts our muscles and connective tissues (the somatic nervous system) to tell us that pleasure or desire is not safe to feel, or that to feel pleasure is to be wrong, or that to feel emotion in sex is to be exposed and open to danger in the presence of another human being. The conflicting nature of what can happen in our bodies during sex can be confounding and frustrating, and the assumptions we then make about this complexity obstructs the fullness of eroticism.

It is possible to learn about what your body truly feels and wants—not the conditioned interpretation that the brain and nervous system has built as a shortcut—while dissolving the judgments that hinder pleasure, connection, and growth. In order to mend the fragmented sexual self and access our erotic potential, we must be able to navigate the terrain of the body in real time. We can then unravel the knots created by cultural pressures on sexuality, unpacking the intellectual and somatic shortcuts at the body level, to reinvigorate the sexual body that has been restricted from new growth. To do so, we need a tool with which to interface with our sexuality, to intelligently explore the interplay between how we relate to our bodies and how our bodies relate to us, to others, and to our environments. That tool is awareness.

The Tools of Refined Awareness

Mindfulness practices are currently riding a strong wave through the fields of psychotherapy, self-help, and even sports and corporate environments. Mindfulness has been found to be effective in the treatment of chronic pain, anxiety, and physical performance and has a growing body of research support. People from all ages and walks of life are learning this powerful awareness practice. First and foremost, mindfulness is a deep listening skill that allows us to make better decisions about how to respond to both internal and environmental stressors. It helps us develop a gap between impulse and action—a moment to breathe and notice before reacting. This allows the body to reveal possibilities in each moment to change the thought and behavioral habits that don't serve us. It also helps us reach a deep, restful state, which can relieve physical and emotional pain. Many hospitals now incorporate mindfulness practice at pain management clinics. At its core, the purpose of mindfulness practice is self-awareness and self-mastery to positively impact our experience of ourselves.

Mindfulness—mind-directed awareness of thoughts and of the body—is just at the surface of how we can access the erotic body. For example, when touring the temple of Apollo at Delphi in Greece, one could look around and utilize the mindfulness skill of identify-what-you-see-without-attachment. "Tree." "Pile of stones." "Warm breeze." This will help you return to the present moment when your mind wanders. Without mindfulness, you may just rely on the tour guide to tell you what you are seeing and quickly move on to the next thing.

What if you notice how your hands want to touch the rocks, or how your front body wants to turn toward the sun to feel its warmth in the early morning coolness, or how your nose compels you to breathe in deeply to smell the pine trees? The temple ruins tell you their story by speaking directly through the gateway of your senses to your bodily experience of sensation, movement impulse, and rhythm as you allow your body to move *with* the temple grounds. It is the awareness of your whole body, the *feeling* impact of being at that particular location, and the real-time way that your body responds to the environment with felt sense and movement action that gives your experience lushness and vibrancy.

It is because of the sensory and movement capacity of the body that our most important experiences in life are written directly into our nervous systems. What we experience organizes us and influences how we respond in the moment and to later life experiences. Mindfulness, while an incredibly valuable tool, lacks the depth to fully encompass the awareness of the whole erotic somatic self. Alternately, the concept of *bodyfulness*, as introduced by somatic psychotherapist and author Christine Caldwell, more clearly and fully articulates what mindfulness practice is trying to attain.

Throughout her many years of writing and practicing as a somatic psychotherapist, Caldwell (2018) has introduced the neologistic term *bodyfulness* to more accurately describe what mindfulness and body-centered practices are ultimately up to—without the Western bias on the importance of the "logical" mind. Bodyfulness, therefore, is a dedicated practice of embedding ourselves in the experience of our body with discipline and nonjudgment in order to "challenge our embodied experience in a way that tempers our compelling and habituated action patterns" (pg. 150).

Bodyfulness is a phenomenological approach to the whole self—a practice that engages the first-person perspective of the whole body or specific areas or systems of the body. What is your quality of breath telling you? The breadth and depth of contraction and release in the muscles and bones of your rib cage are speaking a mother-tongue language to you. They are telling you when they feel safe enough to expand, when they are fatigued (emotionally or physically) and need to rest, or when they are cautious and limiting expansion to take up minimal space and hide. Let these body systems speak directly to you rather than rely on the mind to observe and tell you what it thinks.

When we let the body talk to us, we are less likely to judge or hastily interpret what we find—we are simply listening with a curious ear to what a friend (our own body) is communicating. When we truly listen, we discover the body armor that is initiating the contraction, allowing us to find what is needed in order to soften the defense and move toward pleasure. Perhaps the pelvis tells us it is contracting and shrinking from contact because it wants to be touched in a different way or perhaps the pelvis is not ready to be seen, let alone touched. This becomes an invitation to explore desires, needs, and personal boundaries.

When Erotic Bodyfulness Uncovers Trauma

As psychiatrist and author Bessel van der Kolk (2015) said, "the body keeps the score," and as a result we so often approach sexual connection with ourselves or others from a place of inner conflict and protectiveness. When one has experienced negative sexual moments, including trauma, they are stored in the body by way of the nervous system. This is a normal and healthy response to a threat in the environment as it protects the body and prepares us to deal with a future threat. The difficulty comes when we want to open to a positive sexual experience but this prior response to threat influences how we inhabit the body in the present moment. When sexual stimuli are present, the body memory of trauma activates, and a safe and consensual intimate moment can be experienced as dangerous. Those who have experienced trauma may respond to current sexual situations as traumatic without the awareness that their current stress is based on past wounding.

In sex and sexual expression, the body often attempts to keep safe by retracting from fully experiencing the vulnerable behavior. According to neuroscientist Stephen Porges's polyvagal theory, this is the dorsal-vagal response or Social Inhibitory System being activated because we don't feel safe or because we have negative attributions to what we are experiencing. This is more colloquially referred to as the fight-flight-freeze response.

To apply this directly to sexual intimacy, you'll remember from Chapter 2 that sex educator Emily Nagoski has renamed this the Sexual Inhibition System (SIS). When activated, the SIS inhibits arousal response even when sexually relevant elements are in the immediate environment. Because the body responds to stress by steeling itself against contact with the SIS-activating stimuli from the environment, we cannot open to the pleasure in our body or the arousal detected from a lover. This response can generalize to nonsexual pleasure-inducing activities like dancing or hugging, preventing enjoyment of the many ways we move and express ourselves, especially in relationship with others. The nervous system rapidly sends signals to the heart to quicken its pace, pumping blood away from the core of the body out to the limbs. This process also directs blood away from the pelvis, where blood surrounding the pelvic nerves and tissues is required for sexual arousal. Breathing becomes fast and shallow, pupils dilate to fixate on what feels dangerous, and the stomach tightens to inhibit digestion (an unnecessary use of energy when in danger). Like couriers in a building, the neurochemicals of the nervous system ferry messages from one floor to the next at the pace of lightning, too swiftly to be tracked by consciousness alone. We are now alert and ready to deal with the threat.

But is there really a threat? As a consenting adult who wants to relax this response and let a sexual partner in, how do you call your body back from the SIS response? Bodyfulness practice tunes us into this somatic armoring response in arousal with a whole-body awareness that allows us to slow the rapid escalation of distress, step back into our window of tolerance, and discover pathways of pleasure. By observing the movement and sensations of the body with curiosity, we discover what activated the SIS, and this helps us shift from the SIS (inhibited) to the SES (social engagement/Sexual Excitation System). As we observe and respond to ourselves through bodyfulness practice, we directly contact the split within the sexual self. This split is the polarized remnant of the sociocultural conditioning and negative body memories experienced as an internal incongruence in moments of sexual arousal—pleasure mixed with discomfort, shutdown, or out-of-control behavior.

Interacting with this activation of trauma as a *somatic* experience is a powerful practice that can also be overwhelming. Educator and trauma professional David A. Treleaven identifies the need to recognize that focusing on breath and internal sensations during mindfulness practice can activate panic or dissociation characteristic of having experienced harm or threat to the physical body (2018). Treleaven recommends being on the lookout for a trauma response (intense muscle constriction, lack of muscle tone or "slackness," dissociation, quick and shallow breath) and establishing an anchor of attention as a resource (something that helps you feel grounded that you can return to). For those who have experienced acute or persistent trauma, this work is safer and more effective when explored with trauma-informed support.

Erotic bodyfulness lets you establish a relationship with your natural defenses, allowing the body armor to yield and open the body to deep pleasure, sexual responsiveness, and creativity. Positive psychologist and creativity researcher Mihaly Csikszentmihalyi said in his TED Talk (2014) that "arousal is the area where most people learn from because that is where they are pushed beyond their comfort zone." Erotic bodyfulness aids you in accessing what Csikszentmihalyi defined as the flow state, a space where our abilities are challenged while remaining within the zone of proximal development. This is where our best learning occurs and what many of us have been deprived of within the realm of our developing sexuality.

When bodyfulness is practiced in the erotic realms, it trains the mind to develop a proficiency in the mother-tongue language of the moving, sensory, sexual body. This is the mother-tongue language that we can fully claim as our own. It is not taught to us by anyone in our families or other places in society—it is *innate*. We can reclaim how the body responds to the environment; it is an empowering experience to be able to speak this language and respond congruently. This paves the road to helping us unpack shadows and minimize stereotypes so that we can uncover the truth of wants and desires in real time.

Let's further define this practice of erotic bodyfulness and then focus on the elements that it comprises: present-moment attention, sensation and movement impulse awareness, and internally guided movement sequencing.

Defining Erotic

It is important to be direct about what is meant by *erotic* in the practice of erotic bodyfulness. When I first present this concept to my clients or my workshop participants, I am often initially met with assumptions that account for only a fraction of what is available in the realm of the erotic. In *Uses of the Erotic: The Erotic as Power*, author and activist Audre Lorde (1978, pg. 88) said:

> *The erotic . . . has been made into the confused, the trivial, the psychotic, the plasticized sensation. For this reason, we have often turned away from the exploration and consideration of the erotic as a source of power and information, confusing it with its opposite, the pornographic. But pornography is a direct denial of the power of the erotic, for it represents the suppression of true feeling. Pornography emphasizes sensation without feeling. The erotic is a measure between the beginnings of our sense of self and the chaos of our strongest feelings. It is an internal sense of satisfaction to which, once we have experienced it, we know we can aspire.*

When we listen to the mother-tongue language of the body, we are in the realm of the erotic. Sensation and pleasure can feel good, but the erotic is evoked where pleasure meets with our growing edges and is marked by body tension or recognition of cultural taboos. At this juncture is the clash of the Titans—pleasure and anxiousness, pleasure and pain. Therefore, the erotic turns on the body, the mind, and the ever-evolving soul. It speaks to us of what our deepest personal challenges are, the obstacles to pleasure and fulfillment. The erotic pulls on us from the subterranean depths, mesmerizing us into listening to sensation in all its richness. When the erotic is present, the body flowers open with longing, a compelling drive to push through whatever stands in its way. Like the components found in the rich soil in which we plant our seeds so that they may grow to full bloom, the territory of the erotic invites creativity and expansion. It is nothing less than the potent sexual energy that fuels our creativity and growth, dissolving self-consciousness to evoke full-bodied breath and primal sound.

Ask yourself what elements of an environment inspire you to open yourself to pleasure and connection. When you really listen to what invites your body to open, you may find that erotic elements transcend the candles and soft music setup; your elements could include anything from a warm shower to a leather paddle to a journey through the archetypes of dominant or submissive (the archetypes found within the erotic will be more fully explored in Chapter 8 on mapping the erotic). Everyone has a unique erotic thumbprint, but, unlike your actual thumbprint, what you find erotic may shift and change over your life span.

Enter Erotic Bodyfulness

We can incorporate the practice of bodyfulness into the realm of the erotic to specifically learn about, challenge, and delight in our experiences of pleasure, arousal response, and sexuality in general. In erotic bodyfulness, awareness takes on a primal dimension. Our attention focuses on the bottom-up awareness, the sensory and movement information sent from the body to the mind, from the direct dialogue between the body and the environment (the people, places, and activities) that it finds itself in. This practice focuses on the elements of:

- Sensations like temperature, texture, and inner movement
- Movement impulses and patterns like the gestures, sequences, and posture formed of tension-flow rhythms
- Breath quality (location and depth)
- Use of kinesphere (in what way and how much we take up space) in bipolar or unipolar shape flow patterns

For example, beyond noticing the tension and forward tilt in the pelvis when a lover contacts your genitals, we let the tension in the pelvis say what it wants, what it needs, what way it wants to move. This practice directly validates and allows the nonverbal, mother-tongue language of the body to speak its raw, unfiltered truth. When we slowly follow the lead of body logic, we allow expression to unfold and sequence through. Tension does not stay tense. It may increase in intensity at first, but with breath and movement, the tension unwinds to reveal the deep, aching landscape within.

When bodyfulness is engaged in the erotic realm, we can harness the awareness available from the *whole* body as a sturdy bridge through the inner, unrefined wildness of the erotic with a patient, observant mind. This is a practice that guides us to notice all that is happening in the body with compassion and interest so that we may lean further into what ignites us. We do not have to change who we are or delete painful memories to appreciate our eroticism in the moment; we invite into the foreground the sensations of pleasure without having to forcefully rid ourselves of all discomfort. Erotic bodyfulness keeps us awake to the complex signals of the body and the signals expressed by a lover. It invites an intimacy with the full experience of the self and then the connection with others. What you find within your somatic architecture takes awareness of the mother-tongue language of our sexuality into the action phase.

The Practice

It is time to describe in detail the practice of erotic bodyfulness and provide a road map for how it can be applied. Erotic bodyfulness includes the skills of identifying an "anchor," intentional breath, body awareness (awareness from the whole of the body), oscillating attention, following sensation with description (without judgment or assumption), noticing movement impulse, inviting movement, and following pleasure and yield.

Identify Your Anchor

To begin this practice, identify something that offers you inspiration and allows you to feel safe. Just as Treleaven identified the need for safer mindfulness practice, erotic bodyfulness must include a safeguard to return to when necessary, especially for those who have experienced some form of trauma.

This safeguard is most effective as either an environmental or somatic anchor. An environmental anchor is something in your immediate space that you can see, touch, hear, or smell that you find comforting, grounding, or pleasurable. For example, you may have a favorite rock that you can hold in your hand or an image of a tree full of lights on a summer night that helps you feel safe and present in the moment or can call you back from a troubling memory. You can also request that your lover slow down and tell you that you are safe, loved, or that they love to just be close to you. If you can identify a place in your body that feels comfortable, this somatic anchor can be something to return to when relating with other areas of your body or somatic memories may be challenging.

In addition, somatic trauma therapist Babette Rothschild (2000) recommends "titrating" between the somatic anchor and the somatosensory experience of the body. She likens it to shaking up a bottle of soda and very slowly removing the cap to "off-gas" the emotional distress that may arise. So, once you identify your anchor, practice titrating—shifting your attention back and forth—between your anchor and the sensation that you notice or the movement that you express.

If you have not experienced trauma, you will still benefit from identifying an anchor to help ground and inspire you as you explore your somatic map.

When remembering the language of the body, it is possible to "get lost" in a terrain that may be largely unfamiliar to you. Time and space work differently inside the body and it is possible to feel disoriented at times, especially in the beginning stages of learning this practice.

Intentional Breath

Breath is life, the very spirit that animates our corporal form. This is reflected in our language—both respiration and inspiration share the same Latin root of *spiritus* or *spirit*, meaning *breath*. Breath is that invigorating expansion of the lungs and the alveoli (tiny air sacs that allow for gaseous exchange) within as they fill with the surrounding air, followed by contraction as the air is released. This is the major body system that is unusual in that it is both automatic (breathing happens without conscious thought) and can be directly controlled (we can impact our breath quality at will).

Breathing is a feature of the body that directly embeds us within our environment. We breathe in elements in our environment—most importantly, the oxygen released by trees and plants, which in turn take in the carbon dioxide from our exhale. We also exhale oxygen (about 13%—16%), nourishing others around us. By intentionally widening the rib cage on the in-breath and intentionally relaxing the body and lengthening it during the out-breath, we can slow our heart rate, reduce blood pressure, and invite a sense of letting go in the body as the parasympathetic, the rest-and-digest, nervous system is activated.

I continually invite my clients to "focus on the out-breath" as a means to liberate the tension that is held in their body and therefore make more room for the bodily presence of sensation—both the awareness of sensation and the intensification of it. The breath can also be purposefully guided into other regions of the body to soften the space around body armor, bring awareness to more quiet body regions, and increase sensation by increasing blood and oxygen around the nerve branches of the nervous system. In somatic psychology, we say, "Where breath flows, awareness and sensation go."

Breathing is also one of our most *expressive* body systems. In *The Heart of Yoga* (1995), renowned Viniyoga instructor T. K. V. Desikachar described how inner feelings are expressed through the quality of our breath. Through our breath, these inner feelings influence how we take up space—physical and social—and express how our internal emotions give form to us from within. When we feel safe, our breath expands into the space around us as it takes up more space within our body. Meanwhile, the breath encourages us to shrink into ourselves when we feel anxious or afraid to distance ourselves from the perceived noxious people, things, or activities in our environment. When we tune into the quality of our breath, we notice that it reflects our feeling state (happy, anxious, etc.), and when we *attune*—are aware and receptive—to the quality of another's breath, we can pick up on their emotional state as well. Because breath has the ability to activate awareness in the body and to quickly shift our physical and emotional state, it is a foundational somatic practice and, therefore, the foundation of the practice of erotic bodyfulness.

Erotic Bodyfulness Practice: Intentional Breath

To explore your breath with intention, begin with your eyes closed or a soft gaze if closing your eyes feels like too much. Now place your hand on your chest and invite a full breath in and let a long breath out. Notice how your upper rib cage rises and falls with the breath. Next, place both hands on your lower rib cage/side body and invite the breath again. Notice the increase of distance between your ribs on your in-breath and decrease space on your out-breath. Lean your back into your chair or other surface and press your spine into the surface behind you on your in-breath and soften your back muscles into the cushion on your out-breath. My somatic psychotherapy teacher and mentor Leah D'Abate taught me to visualize a tiny pair of lungs within every cell of the body and then expand every cell on the in-breath. Softening your mouth as you punctuate the out-breath, like fogging a mirror in front of your mouth, can catalyze a fuller release in your jaw, shoulders, and pelvis. Try softening your jaw and pelvic muscles simultaneously on your out-breath, opening the vertical central corridor of breath in your body. Through this central corridor, from throat to pelvic floor, let your breath bubble up like water rising in a fountain to the crown of your head. Then, on the out-breath, allow the breath to release like the water cascading from the top of the fountain down into the pool of your pelvis below. As sensation increases, breath (and later, movement) can also aid you in guiding sensation deeper into your body and from one region to another.

To access the erotic with the breath, notice the warmth of your hand on your body and "listen" for the places where your body is communicating elements of pleasure. Then let your breath help to expand the vicinity of pleasure, expanding the pleasurable sensations into surrounding areas on the in-breath and yielding into these areas on the out-breath. Pleasure can be anything that feels good, not just what we would initially describe as sexual pleasure. Pleasure could be a sensation of warmth, softness, tingling, fluttering, etc. Let each in-breath guide the pleasurable sensation into ever more regions of your inner landscape.

Whole-Body Awareness

Body awareness is not simply about the mind's awareness of the body, but about the awareness that can be found and refined as the inner landscape of your body becomes more aware itself. Every area and system of the body has the ability of awareness. It speaks in the mother-tongue language of sensation, movement, and interdependent exchange with the whole of your body. This is because your body is embedded within the environment via the exteroceptive and interoceptive senses throughout the nervous system. We are most familiar with the awareness of the mind, but the awareness of body systems has gained recognition through research in neuroscience and in the medical field.

For example, the gut-brain connection has been extensively documented by gastroenterologists and neuroscientists, and the gut—stomach and intestines—has been referred to as the *belly brain*. The stomach and intestines are lined with millions of nerve cells, which send signals to the rest of the body about how the gut is feeling. This connection can impact sensations, mood, and behavior long before the conscious mind can catch on to those things. Digestive systems also have awareness and speak to us in the language of peristalsis (waves of muscle contraction traveling through the digestive tract), bubbles, mood fluctuations, and other belly movements. Lungs have awareness and communicate this awareness to us in the form of breath quality, as discussed earlier. Body-centered sex therapist Stella Resnick identifies that the genitals have an erotoceptive awareness that speaks to us in the form of engorgement of erectile tissues, temperature, moisture, pleasure, pain, constriction, softness, and so much more.

By combining body awareness and breath in erotic bodyfulness practice, we can locate the sensations that are pleasurable and amplify them, contain them, and connect to the wisdom that pleasure offers. The wisdom of pleasure tells us about what the body wants to expand toward—what the body is curious about and interested in exploring further. Ultimately, this practice makes us aware of the internal landscape of arousal which is, at its essence, the expansive language of pleasure. I will talk extensively about arousal in the next chapter.

Erotic Bodyfulness Practice: Awareness of the Whole Body

The practice of tuning into the awareness of your whole body begins by scanning the inner and outer landscape of your body for the sensations of texture, temperature, movement, tightness, and openness. Again, you may have your eyes closed or a soft gaze depending on what helps you to remain grounded and curious during your exploration. When you find sensation in each area, pause, and take another full in-breath and out-breath, letting the breath pool like water in each area. You are in no hurry to scan quickly; instead, move slowly and take your time. As you detect sensation, speak in the present tense, using the first person ("I")—speak the awareness of that area of the body directly. For example, if you find an achy constriction in your throat that feels like a vise grip, say "I am vise-grip constricting." Or if you notice a tingly warmth throughout your belly, say, "I am tingling warmth." Notice what happens in your body in response after each awareness. Placing awareness and speaking the language of the body will have an impact.

Now, sit or stand in a comfortable position and invite a full-body in-breath and let the out-breath release strongly with a "ha!" sound. Repeat this three times and let your breath return to normal. Notice your facial muscles, where they are contracted and where they are soft and open. Notice the sensation in and around your throat and neck, the experience at the gateway between your spine and the base of your skull. What are the sensations in your shoulders, down the muscles surrounding the column of your spine? Breathe down through your arms, hands, and fingers. What sensations do you notice traveling between your shoulders to your fingertips? What do you notice in your chest, around your heart, and at the threshold of your diaphragm and solar plexus? Breathe around your belly. What sensations do you notice around your stomach, other abdominal organs, and intestines? Breathe into your pelvic bowl. What sensations do you notice in your pelvis, your genitals, your pelvic floor? Scan your legs and feet. What do you notice through your thigh muscles, knees, shins, ankles, tops of the feet, between the bones of your feet, and the soles of your feet?

At each area, notice how the simple act of awareness changes the sensory experience. After you pause and breathe at each location, ask yourself, "Does it feel the same or is it different?"

Oscillating Attention

Awareness is multifaceted attention. To oscillate is to move back and forth between multiple things—between the many sites of body awareness, between the internal landscape of the body and the surface of the skin, between self and other, between one point in space (narrow attention) and a panoramic attention that takes in multiple elements at once—all at a variable pace. This oscillation has a quality of a nonjudgmental and multiple-perspective way of being. It encourages us to not get fixated on inhibiting discomfort or on enhancing pleasure. Fixation triggers rigidity, increasing narrowness and unconscious behavior. Oscillating attention will allow you to deepen arousal instead of quickening it. As you oscillate your awareness, begin to engage what somatic psychotherapist Leah D'Abate calls "one eye in, one eye out." Or, in other words, the oscillation maintains awareness of one area of the body while inviting the awareness of another area to notice the interrelationship of these two areas as well as the impact of sensation in one area of the body on another. You can also oscillate awareness between your body and someone or something outside of the self.

Erotic Bodyfulness Practice: Oscillate Attention

Practice oscillating between the numerous sites of awareness in your body. Close your eyes or have a soft, unfixed gaze. Begin oscillating somatic awareness while you are doing something you love to do (gardening, playing guitar, being sexual, etc.) and bring your awareness to your breath, how your rib cage expands and contracts. Then, with your out-breath, soften your mouth and shift to the awareness in the position of your body—what is your posture and position telling you about how you are inhabiting the space? Oscillate awareness between chest/ heart space and belly, then belly and pelvis/genitals, then pelvis and back body/spine and back muscles, then facial muscles and jaw, making sure to listen at each body site. With each oscillation, allow your breath and awareness to pool around the areas.

As you oscillate between different areas, can you begin to feel the pathways between them, how they are quite literally connected? Take note of the thoughts that appear in your mind as you visit these body sites and networks and then return to listening to the mother-tongue language arising from these sites. Practice gently dislodging your awareness when it gets stuck in one place. Arousal is compelling and can take a hold of attention toward a desire or goal, so oscillate between narrow attention (focusing on one thing) to panoramic attention (taking in multiple things at once, like the dynamic or system created by you and a lover).

Follow Sensation With Description

As you oscillate with intentional breath from one point of sensation to many points of sensation, and from your internal to external environment, see if you can keep returning to *description* rather than interpretation. This means that you stay with the present-moment sensation and move away from judgment, assumption, stereotype, and interpretation. When you practice erotic bodyfulness and you find yourself thinking "Ugh, my back hurts again; I'm getting old," shift your awareness away from the judgment and back into describing the experience, such as "In this moment, my back hurts . . . I am a dull, aching cylinder down the sides of my spine." Invite a full breath around the area and ask your spine what it needs to feel supported. Then follow the guidance of the body—a tilt of the pelvis, a pillow behind your back, lying with your back to the floor. When you feel the dull ache lessen, ask yourself "What is here now?" and flow your awareness to a place in your body where you feel good (which may be your back after you address the discomfort). Observing and relating to your body from a place of description instead of interpretation allows a gentle yet radical dismantling of what we have assumed to be true about our body and our sexuality. The inhibiting sexual schemas, gender schemas, and relational schemas begin to unravel when what we believed to be true turns out to be much more complex and richer on the level of sensation.

Erotic Bodyfulness Practice: Follow Sensation With Description

As you scan your somatic landscape and oscillate your attention between areas, notice when you take on a judgmental or critical tone. Perhaps you have a body discomfort or injury that is the loudest sensation during your practice and you find yourself saying "This pain is preventing me from doing the real work!" or "I shouldn't be focusing on that right now—I'm supposed to be focusing on erotic sensations, dammit!" Notice the impact of this judgmental tone on your somatic self. Chances are that your body further closes to your awareness. You have activated your own body armor, protecting yourself from your own unkind words. Instead, return to description to validate your experience. "The back of my thigh speaks of electric pain." Or "My nose speaks of an itching and tingling into release with a sneeze." What is frustrating or annoying to us becomes a part of the process. How you speak to your body during this practice, no matter what sensation shows up, defines the quality of relationship that you are cultivating with your body.

Next, if you find yourself describing sensation with words like "good," "excited," or "sad," do not be content with these umbrella terms. Take the time to describe in detail the qualities of the feeling. A feeling of excitement perhaps becomes "a bouncing tingle between my solar plexus and throat." A "fleshed-out" description allows you to access the feeling body as subject instead of object—a first-person account spoken by the excitement instead of a narration by your thoughts.

Notice Movement Impulse

As you continually return to listening to the mother tongue of the body, you may notice an emergent impulse for movement. In contrast to being "impulsive," noticing a movement *impulse* (from the Latin *impellere*, to push or drive) is to detect the inception of internal motion. This stage of the practice finds the origin points of your expression—the micro-movements felt through interoceptive (internal sense) awareness. You will find that these micro-movement impulses are in continual dance throughout the spaces where your nervous system weaves into your soft tissues, muscles, and organs. For example, movement impulses can be utilitarian ("I notice an impulse from my dry mouth to reach for my drink or from my cold arms to reach for a blanket"), safety oriented ("I notice an impulse from my side body to shrink away from a person who is yelling at me"), or relational ("I notice an impulse to soften into a lover from my chest area").

Using dance/movement therapy, I encourage my clients to slowly follow these uncovered movement impulses in session, to exaggerate the movement, or to involve more or fewer areas of the body in the movement. This form of movement exploration invites the discovery of what feels familiar, learning the habituated patterns of movement, or body memories almost frozen in time. This type of movement exploration also allows the unlocking of a broader movement repertoire; a movement impulse could be a new action and movement option surfacing as a result of exploration. This broader movement repertoire could be movements that you wanted to make in the past but couldn't, action sequences that you could not follow, or movements that you made that you did not want to.

Erotic Bodyfulness Practice: Notice Movement Impulse

As you focus on the present moment with eyes closed or a soft gaze, you may notice openness or warmth in one area of the body and constriction in another part of the body. Ask yourself, what is the warmth in my chest telling me? What is the constriction in my pelvis telling me? What do they need to find congruence? As you move both breath and awareness into the constriction of the pelvis, the sensation may begin to shift and give you a clue to what is needed—more breath or softened jaw and shoulders. Your pelvis may need to know that it is safe to open, it is safe to breathe, it is worthy of attention. Listen closely and pause before following the movement impulse. The potential energy of a movement impulse is dense with emotional and psychological material. Surround the impulse with breath and take the time to listen before moving on.

Invite Movement From the Impulse

As a kid, I used to play "still as a statue" and loved the feeling of holding as still as I possibly could in a sudden and awkward body position. I could feel the excited tension building in my muscles as I waited to be released from the game leader. It is clear during this game that we are never truly still. Even though you may be sitting still, your body is continually moving. As I stood as still as a statue, I felt my heart pump, the micro-movements of my muscles contracting and releasing in a coordinated effort to keep me in some awkward vertical position, my dry eyes longing to blink. As you read this, notice the involuntary micro-movements in the muscles of your face, the subtle shifts in your seat, the slight wiggle of your toes. Notice the expansion and contraction of the rib cage with your breath. Turn on a piece of music with a beat and notice how your body automatically responds to the rhythm, swaying and tapping your foot as if being taken over by a pair of magical dancing shoes. Like all living creatures, the human body is in constant motion. By detecting the presence of the micro-movements of the body as discussed in the *notice movement impulse* section earlier, you can slowly invite these movements to get bigger and more gestural.

These subtle micro-movements are the building blocks of larger movement patterns—habitual, adaptive, responsive, and expressive. Dancer, director, and choreographer Alvin Ailey said, "Each movement is the sum total of moments and experiences." By itself, a micro-movement is just a twitch of the eye or flex of the finger, but when accumulated, we discover composite body patterns rich with information about how we have adapted to experience and express ourselves in relationship. These composite movement patterns, or inner landscapes, unlock body and cognitive memories, stored emotions, and even imagery, which reflects to us the larger meaning of what our body needs to say.

To illustrate: Olivia is a white, 52-year-old paralegal who started working with me because her interest in sexual pleasure had been nonexistent for many years. More than a lack of desire, Olivia described a lack of sensation in her pelvis and vulva. She feared that her sexuality was "dead." We explored her body history and Olivia reported no physical injuries that could cause her pelvic nerve to be pinched and no scar tissue in her arousal or reproductive anatomy that could deaden sensation or cause pain. We also explored her touch history and found no overt physical or sexual abuse, just a loving upbringing within a low-touch family. Over the course of her relationship with a sexual partner from college, Olivia had continually agreed to sex while her body continually said a clear "no," tightening and recoiling on a micro-level against her partner's touch. As I invited Olivia to find and slowly follow the movement impulse of the "no," her torso hollowed, shoulders wrapped around like rigid sentinels, and her hands formed a wall in front of her pelvis. As she slowly repeated this movement with an increasingly stronger out-breath, her "no" became a loud, burning thrust away from her body. "I'm so mad that I made myself have sex when I didn't want to," she began. "I just wanted to keep the peace because I loved my partner." Olivia finally released tears from her anger as I reflected, "You don't have to do anything you don't want to." Then, "What do you notice now?" I asked, prompting her to listen to the awareness of her inner landscape as we had practiced in our work. Olivia slowly looked up at me, eyes wide, and said, "I am feeling relief in my chest, like a soft waterfall . . . and I notice warmth and tingling in my pelvis!" Olivia's arousal anatomy sensation had been uncovered!

Intentionally moving with movement impulses is the foundational practice of what dance/movement therapy utilizes to uncover what is called *authentic movement*. Mary Whitehouse said that it is the found movement of the body that can liberate us. Intentionally following and clarifying the quality and trajectory of the impulses that precede automatic movement allows our adaptive schemas to unfold. We can, along the pathway of the movement, notice where we naturally impede the unfolding of a need or desire as we notice the corresponding self-talk. Follow the movement that your body wants, and you will have the opportunity to soften the body armor defense as clearer and more satisfying movement develops.

Slow and intentional movement supports understanding of what is needed to continue to follow the original impulse (before it became a habitual movement response) as well as knowledge of how to generate effective personal action in relationships. This allows your body to express its deepest needs and therefore open the gates to deeper experience and expression. Also, both micro-movements and larger movements increase oxygen and blood flow in the body, which in turn enhances sensation and further unlocks feeling potential, allowing us to follow our pleasure.

Erotic Bodyfulness Practice: Invite Movement From the Impulse

Like the "still as a statue" game I used to play as a kid, invite your body into stillness so that the subtler micro-movements can begin to front-load your awareness. Soften your gaze or close your eyes and invite three full breaths. Scan your internal landscape for sensation until you locate a movement impulse. Allow your breath and awareness to pool like water around the origin point of movement, noticing the direction and quality of movement that it wants to initiate. Slowly follow this movement impulse, letting it guide you to its conclusion—move until the movement feels complete. Now, exaggerate and repeat the movement impulse until it becomes a clear and purposeful sequence of motion. Gently dislodge your awareness from thoughts or assumptions about the unfolding movement and return to the awareness of your moving body. Ask yourself:

- *Does this feel familiar?*
- *What need is this movement trying to accomplish?*

- *Do I have an image arising?*
- *What do I notice now that I have explored this movement impulse?*
- *What is the next movement impulse that I notice?*

Follow Pleasure and Yield

As you breathe with sensation and follow movement impulses, charting the hills and valleys until a pattern and landscape emerge, you begin to form a somatic erotic map. What once seemed random becomes cumulative and cohesive. Think of pleasure as rivers flowing around and between rocks of tension or numbness. Over time, the persistent water softens the edges of the rocks, just as Olivia discovered and moved her anger with clear purpose to open to tingling and warmth in her pelvis, ultimately opening the door to pleasure once again.

Once Olivia had followed the "no" movement and released her anger, she was able to locate the internal movement impulse to soften. As her pelvis filled with blood and oxygen at long last, the pleasure that emerged became the new impulse for movement. Olivia stood in my office and followed the swirls that formed throughout her vulva and womb area, slowly moving in circles and figure eights to find the movement pathway that supported the expansion of the warmth and tingling. Through the circles and undulations with her breath, she felt the warmth expand into her belly, creating butter-flies, and rise like arching wings through her spine and over her shoulders. She repeated the undulation from her pelvis as it gradually extended her torso and guided her arms to rise over her head in a sweeping motion. I reflected to Olivia her full butterfly form, light and warm. In this moment, Olivia recalled the mastery with which she swam through the water with her butterfly stroke as a young woman. Olivia laughed, delighted that this was a place that she knew all along yet, until this moment, had never connected with her eroticism. I watched as the muscles around her eyes became smooth and she rested into her back body, a relaxed smile on her lips. Olivia had com-pleted the pleasure sequence and now yielded into the softness of her body.

Over the course of our work, Olivia continually referred to this session as her turning point. She felt a somatic and imagery shift in her experience of her own body and, in moments of her body armor returning, she had a move-ment pathway to reclaim this butterfly-like somatic experience. Once she had reclaimed her whole-body "no" with confidence in her personal boundaries, this allowed her to access her whole-body "yes." In order to keep this resilient pleasure movement sequence going, Olivia even took up swimming again. Every time she enters the water, she finds the origin point of a pleasurable movement impulse and follows it through the water until she feels the yield response.

In this context, to yield into your body is not about conceding to defeat; it is an active and intentional softening into the experience of your body. No longer fighting against sensation or movement, the yield is the agreement to truly open your senses and listen to discomfort, pleasure, or whatever is showing up in each moment.

Erotic Bodyfulness Practice: Follow Pleasure and Yield

Soften your gaze or close your eyes as you invite three full breaths, scan your body for sensation, notice a movement impulse and follow it. As you uncover places of pleasure, use your breath and the movement impulse found within the site of your pleasure to slowly and intentionally circulate it to other areas of your body. Follow a movement impulse and then invite a deep out-breath as you relax into the moment and yield into your body, awaiting the next impulse. For example, if you feel pleasure in your pelvis and tension in your belly, guide your breath to expand your belly and draw the sensation of pleasure upward toward your diaphragm area and downward toward your legs. The sensation and movement pathways form the inner erotic map that exists within you, ever evolving.

Repeat the pleasurable movement until you begin to feel a softening, an invitation to yield. Now, invite your body back into stillness and feel the inner movements of pleasure continuing to cycle within even as you sit quietly.

Putting It All Together

Obviously, we probably won't start this work as a full butterfly. More often, we begin this work weighed down by frustration or fear or self-criticism, yet still searching. Erotic bodyfulness (see Figure 4.1), when practiced with diligence and persistence, can rewrite habitual body patterns that keep us locked in an erotic stockade. We are well practiced at our external and critical focus and we are rewarded for this in many areas of life, from academia to business. This is the *yield* into a different space of receptivity and alertness.

As you apply this practice to your experience, you may not make it through all seven steps every time. Let me be clear: this is not meant to be practiced in the same order and through every step, every time. You may begin by practicing intentional breathing with awareness from different areas of your body, oscillating and yielding, with no detectable movement or pleasure arising. Or you may find yourself engaging in a movement that suddenly feels interesting as you engage body awareness, followed by an intentional breath

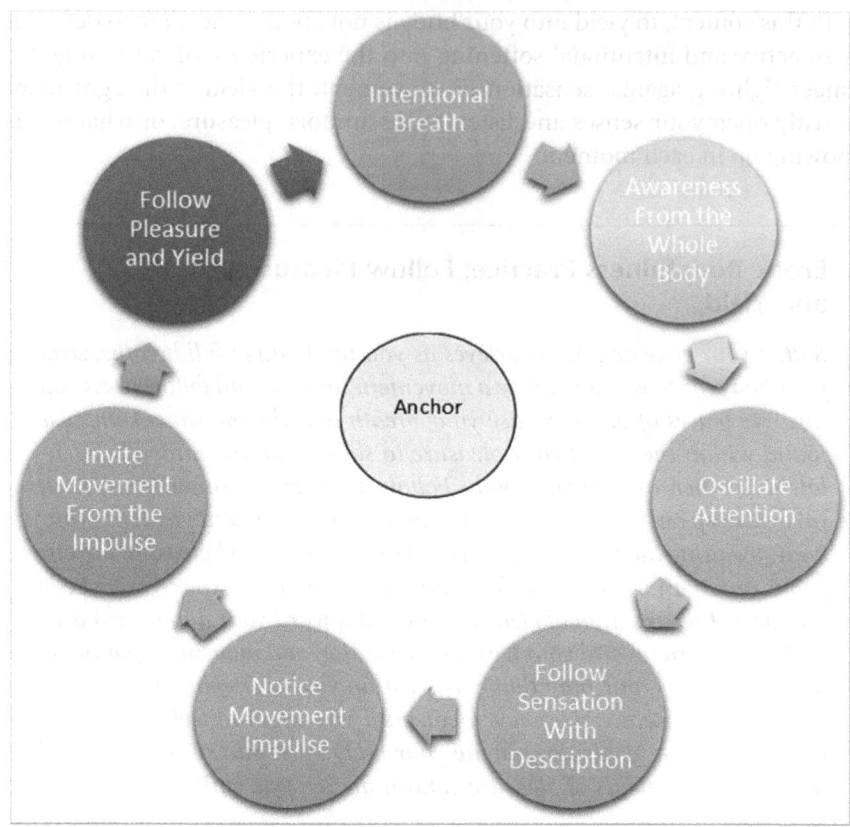

Figure 4.1 Erotic Bodyfulness Sequence

to stabilize and deepen your sensation. You may arrive at the moment of noticing a movement impulse only to have self-criticism take hold of you, jolting you away from your intentional breath and connection with sensation. Don't worry. This is all part of the practice. Dislodge your attention from the critical thoughts and return to step one—intentional breath—and begin the practice again. Each fundamental step benefits from repetition and mastery. In other words, you'll get better at this over time. My partner, who is a Brazilian jiujitsu (BJJ) coach, encourages all BJJ practitioners to "return to the fundamentals because there is always a deeper understanding to be found there"—even by those who hold the highest belt and mastery levels.

Once you arrive at the point where you can follow your movement impulses and find pleasure, continue the slow and thoughtful pace of your awareness to merge all seven steps into each moment. When these seven steps can be woven into each moment of erotic bodyfulness practice, you may experience a flow state—a seamless state of "moving and being moved."

Erotic Bodyfulness in the Nonsexual Realm

Bodyful sex can be a difficult concept to introduce. I find that it is helpful to start this practice where we feel *safe enough* to venture. Many of my clients find that beginning with sex when learning the practice of erotic bodyfulness is daunting because sex is their primary source of stress and anxiety when they first come to see me, especially if they have a history of sexual trauma.

When my clients are frustrated with the responsiveness of their body in sex or are struggling with a lack of desire for sex, I first invite them to widen their lens to find where their erotic energy *is* flowing freely—where they already experience the somatosensory presentation of pleasure. At its essence, erotic or sexual energy shows up as the rhythm of intensity rising into a peak followed by a release in the body—a sensory wave building and washing over us. In dance/movement therapy, this is the *surging and birthing* rhythm—a "building up to an intense pressure in the effort of creation, and then followed by a strong but gradual release" (Kestenberg-Amighi, Loman, & Sossin, 2018, pg. 49). This rhythm can be felt in the genitals, the gut, the heart, and the mind and has the ability to flow through the whole body—and can be found in both sexual and nonsexual realms.

So, we begin by identifying where clients feel *safe enough* AND *excited enough* to feel the effortless wave of this generative energy. The rhythmic pleasure response of the body is found in more configurations and places than our general understanding of the human sexual response gives us credit for. *Sexual energy always finds a way*. It may not be in the bedroom at first, but we all experience it *somewhere*. My work with clients takes a panoramic lens, scanning all corners of their life and their somatic map for the evidence of pleasurable experience and connection.

As a dancer, I intimately know the experience of walking into the studio with cold muscles, warming up my body with movement, finding a flow with the music and perhaps other dancers, reaching a peak moment of whole-body euphoria, followed by my body naturally returning to a place of rest and reflection. In my dance sessions, I notice a building of pleasure in my body, a moving through a physical challenge, and a transformative moment or moments on which to later reflect. This is personal somatic research on responsiveness to pleasure—the study and celebration of sensual and sexual wellness. Once a pleasurable activity is found, the embodied research begins. Bringing the skill of erotic bodyfulness online, awareness is slowed and interoception begins. By recognizing that we can access places from which to feel and express more fully, we build a knowing of pleasure and a resource to return to when we venture into the shadow realms of our sexuality.

A white, queer-identified, 26-year-old graduate student, Martin, struggled with feeling "claustrophobic" when his partner initiated sex. He found the practice of erotic bodyfulness during partner intimacy a real challenge. When I explored other places where Martin could access pleasure with a sense of spaciousness, he brightened almost immediately. "Even before I get into the hot tub at the end of a long day, I'm already looking forward to it. I can feel my muscles aching for the release. And when I finally get in . . . whew!—what a release! It's like an orgasm in my muscles as soon as I sink into the hot water," he laughed. Martin found his buildup and release in an unlikely—and just as satisfying—place. In session, I guided Martin through the seven layers of erotic bodyfulness as he visualized submerging his body in the hot tub. He found an effortless quality to accessing intentional breath, following movement impulses, and the sensation of pleasure emerged in his body. As homework, I invited him to continue this practice while actually in the hot tub, sequencing through the flowy arm movements and upper-body sway that he had played out during our session.

Martin returned to session the following week having thoroughly enjoyed this experience. "Even better," he said, "I practiced in the shower and during that thunderstorm we had last weekend. I *am* a Pisces, so it makes sense that water in general can give me that bodygasm that you talked about!"

I then invited Martin to stand in my office and, while visualizing his time in the water, begin to move his body directly from the source of sensation that arose. As his arms sequenced a flowy movement from his hips and spine out through his arms and fingertips, I asked what sensations he noticed. "Rippling . . . warmth . . . expanding," he said. As he continued his movements, eyes closed and with a deeply inward focus with the erotic bodyfulness practice, I invited him to say, "My sexuality is rippling, my sexuality is warmth, my sexuality is expanding"—using the very words his body had already given us. He slowly spoke the words aloud as his breath deepened. His shoulders and facial muscles softened as he, so subtly, yielded into himself. "Ahhhhhh," he sounded on the out-breath. "This is your truth," I said to him. When he opened his eyes, he became giddy. He had experienced another side to his sexuality—not just claustrophobic or constricted. His erotic map was actually vast and inviting. Eventually, Martin invited his partner into the hot tub with him and, as he connected with his watery eroticism, he was delighted to feel his body respond in a receptive and interested way to his partner's touch.

A Path to Savoring the Erotic

The path to savoring the erotic requires learning how to bring our attention inward and then outward to things in the environment that we find erotic, oscillating our attention to embrace our full experience, moment to moment. By shifting our awareness back and forth between the many-faceted internal and external realms, we are less likely to get stuck in self-consciousness or a painful memory. Shame, resentment, anger, and a sense of rejection often surface when we believe that our desires must be suppressed. This practice allows us to enjoy, explore, and circulate arousal energy instead of forcing ourselves to just get through it or shutting off and sequestering arousal when faced with internalized familial or societal judgment or prior challenging sexual experiences.

Everything we explore in relationship to sexuality is referred back to the inner landscape of the body, the interoceptive senses telling us of our inner experience of sensation. When we explore our sexual behaviors, we notice how they impact our somatic self. When we explore our experience and expression of gender identity, we notice our somatic self. When we explore arousal anatomy—the sexual response cycle, beliefs, values, or desires of a partner—we notice our somatic self. When talking to a client who holds a long-assumed belief that solo sex (masturbation) is dirty, I might ask: do you notice both a pleasure response and a tightness in the chest and stomach? What is the pleasure response connected to? What is the tightness response connected to? Let these two seemingly opposing internal responses have a conversation. What does each response want? Or what is a response protecting you from? It is within the internal landscape that the unlearning and relearning begins.

We often take these bodily responses for granted and because it feels bad or confusing, *we further distance ourselves from ourselves*. With any aspect of sexuality, erotic bodyfulness practice gives us the skill to be in the present moment with our internal experience. This is what keeps us in real-time awareness as we explore the complex levels of sexuality in a socialized context. Learning to understand and speak the language of the body is *the* core component of this perspective—in the words of professor and youth activist Ramon Parish in a class lecture, "We no longer swallow our culture whole." We develop a one-to-one relationship with ourselves that is characterized by compassion, curiosity, and permission—all the characteristics that can be socialized out of us. Now we are able to discern between the threads within us that weave together to create our emergent sexuality.

5

THE WHOLE SEXUAL SELF

*B*reathe. Fill your chest, belly, and pelvis with a fresh in-breath. Allow your muscles to settle in over your bones on the out-breath. Soften the muscles around your face and allow your gaze to gently rest on the page in front of you. Now, submerge your whole pelvis with breath, allowing the pelvic muscles to give, gently expanding on the in-breath and resting into the seat beneath you on the out-breath. If you notice thoughts, release them with a softening of your eyes and return to the landscape of your body. Breathe in the words "I am safe, I am beautiful, I am whole." If emotion arises, let it move through you with your breath and adjustment in your seat. Let your chin rest a little closer to your chest and be right here in this moment.

Return your awareness to your pelvis and breathe around your arousal and reproductive anatomy—your erectile tissue (all genders have a similar amount), your nerve networks, your soft tissues, and the muscular bowl of your pelvis. Oscillate your attention up into your belly, solar plexus, and chest. What sensations do you notice? Tightness, bubbling, fluttering, warmth, coldness, numbness? Breathe around your pelvis, torso, and jaw all at once. Can you find the pathway that traverses your pelvis through your torso into your jaw? By way of nerve networks and connective tissues, this gorgeous pathway is there, interweaving the whole of your body. Allow your awareness of this pathway to deepen and evolve. Try ever so slowly tilting your pelvis forward, connecting the whole base of your pelvis with the seat beneath you. Notice how the movement sequences from your pelvis and waist into your spine and upper body as your body accommodates such a small movement.

Now slowly, slowly tilt your pelvis backward, curling and lowering your center of gravity. Allow your out-breath to follow the downward movement of your torso and lower your chin to your chest. Now alternate tilting your

DOI: 10.4324/9780429297236-6

pelvis forward, breathing into your arousal anatomy and noticing the sequence of movement to lift you up, and tilting your pelvis backward, softening your arousal anatomy and noticing the sequence of movement to lower your upper body into your seat. Repeat as many times as you like. You are elegantly interwoven, from your sexual organs, through the corridor of your body, to your jaw, mouth, and mind. Breathe into your whole self as one.

This is the sort of reparative experience—a whole-body inclusive way of conceptualizing and experiencing your arousal anatomy and sexual responsiveness—that is needed to rewrite the years of unhelpful, inaccurate, and fragmenting information that so many of us take in. As this new paradigm is presented in the following pages, I invite you to reclaim a complex and inclusive sexual self. My hope is that you fall in love with your body—your own arousal anatomy and sexual responsiveness—and discover the sexual health within you, with both your expressiveness and defenses included. The integrated sexual self gives you the information you need to heal the distrust and frustration that develops as a sexual being in your family, peer groups, and, more broadly, society or culture. Through discovery and learning, we refine the erotic body's pleasure, expressiveness, and responsibility.

While opening to the pleasure of being in a body, it is necessary to tend to the parts of the sexual self that have been boxed, mislabeled, and neglected—where the social and cultural shadows have inflicted harm and distortion. This is helpful when dismantling the antiquated sex-as-performance and sex-as-natural paradigms. According to psychologist Carol Rinkleib Ellison, "The sex-as-performance model presupposes that sex should just happen 'naturally' with little forethought or active planning" (Kleinplatz, 2012, pg. 141). The old paradigm of sexual response that supports the beliefs that underpin sex-as-performance—the medicalized, fear-based, and norm-based approach to the erotic body—has highjacked so many people with its narrow understanding and experience of pleasure and connection.

The impersonal presentation of stand-alone genital functions and reproductive systems is alienating—we are often told to dismiss the way that the pelvis is intimately woven into the whole body. In reality, the sexual and reproductive systems are elegantly interconnected with the nervous system, and therefore impacted by the senses, the emotional body, the mind, and the impact of relationships and environments. Yet we are so often encouraged to feel both separate from, and critical of, the sexual self.

This limiting perspective labels many points along the normal range of sexuality as suspect and problematic. It also disregards the intimate and emotional nature inherent in relating to the erotic body. Holistic sex educator Sheri Winston (2010) says that "along with all the overt messages about how cool it is to be young and hip, and how hot it is to look and act sexy, we get contrary and more covert message that tells us actual sex is shameful and embarrassing" (pg. 24). When we have early negative experience learning about or experiencing our arousal anatomy (so many of us do), we could hear just the word "sex" and our amygdala activates, readying our defensive strategies. Like a call to arms in the brain, the amygdala links perceived threat with our survival response and we drop into a rapid series of preset actions to deal with the threat. With increased amygdala activity, we are bathed in the stress hormone cortisol and the prefrontal cortex—the part of the brain that houses the executive functions of perspective and problem-solving— goes off-line (Cozolino, 2017). As a result, our body armor is activated and impacts our experience in the relational space. Lacking total body connectivity and congruence within the sexual self, responses are rigid, disjointed, and incongruent. When we acknowledge the prevalence of body-shaming and negative attitudes toward pleasure, it makes sense that most people would lose focus at the mere mention of the penis or vagina. Why else would snickering be the most common response to sex talk? Humor diverts our attention from discomfort and releases tension.

Unfortunately, this old paradigm is not just an outdated textbook that we can laugh off as archaic and promptly toss into the recycling bin. If that were the case, learning an embodied perspective on arousal anatomy would be as simple as picking up a freshly updated version of sexuality to read and put directly into practice. In actuality, as a result of the experience-dependent construction of the nervous system, we incorporate the negative tone, the rigid and breath-vacant body posture of our cultural sexuality representatives on a deeply implicit, somatic level. While one quarter of the memory may be consciously recalled as an overt memory, three quarters of the memory is stored implicitly, below conscious awareness in our muscles and movement responses. In other words: we relate with the world from a sex-negative foundation without realizing it.

After several months of working together, Andrew and Brittany started their weekly session talking about their frustration with how they responded to their ten-year-old son's questions about sex. "We both feel that sex is a positive thing and we are excited about the work we are doing as a couple," Brittany, a white, 33-year-old from a conservative Italian-American family in Boston, begins. The muscles around her eyes contract as she says, tightness in her voice, "so why was I so flustered when Jack asked me what a condom was?!" Brittany and Andrew talked about trying to stay open with Jack as they described what contraception is. Meanwhile, they both reported tightness in their chest and shakiness in their breath. "I wanted so badly to give him this information in a more positive way than I did as a kid," Andrew's long out-breath collapsed his shoulders and hollowed his chest. Andrew, a black, middle-aged man from Georgia, received a similarly fear-based sex education from his conservative Catholic school years. I assured them that, due to their early negative learning experiences about sex, their internal defense systems were a normal response. We spent the session practicing asking and answering questions about sex as I cheered them on. We laughed together, shared a few tears, and both left the session feeling more confident that they could bring the topic up with their son and more comfortably discuss his important curiosities.

Our learning of sexuality is deeply unconscious and our responses are reflexive. What is written on our nervous system internally becomes expressed externally, whether we want it to or not. Brittany and Andrew both expressed what dance artist and theorist Rudolf Laban called *shadow movements*— the automatic movements made by our bodies that reveal the truth of what we feel.

To truly reintegrate sexuality with the whole of your being, we must untangle the toxic threads from the healthy ones and reweave ourselves into a holistic tapestry. As you read this chapter, you will be invited to make note of these toxic strands as they begin to unravel. You will also be invited to explore the pleasure strands as they arise and begin to move more freely within your body. In later chapters, I will discuss even more fully the expressive component of this process. But for now, let's begin with writing.

Erotic Bodyfulness Practice

- *Writing: Describe your memory of learning about sex, arousal anatomy, and reproductive anatomy. Did you learn formally, as in health class at school? Did you learn informally at home? What were the explicit (stated clearly and in detail) messages that you received? What were the implicit (inferred and nonverbal) messages that you detected?*
- *Interoception: As you write, turn your attention to your breath. What is the current rate and depth of your breath? Explore your internal sensations as though they form a topographic map. Do you notice tightness in your muscles? What other sensations do you notice? What posture do you find yourself in? What is your body telling you about your experience through sensation and movement?*

A New Paradigm of Sexual Wellness

Now for the good news. The erotic body can be accessed no matter our life circumstances, our level of physical ability, whether or not we have children, whether we have stressful jobs, whether we live with illness or disability, and even whether or not we have experienced trauma. These circumstances create challenges—challenges that can be engaged with on a somatic level to broaden the erotic map beyond the narrow sexual scripts we are given. The erotic body is where valuable, personal learning and evolution can take place. The key is not measuring ourselves against the external, perceived standard. Instead, we look inward and follow the warm, red thread of pleasure to its source—a road that winds through and around obstacles and into wide-open spaces. The secret that I tell my clients is that even when they do not fit into their perception of normative sociocultural windows of "normal" or "ideal" sexual functioning, they do experience healthy sexuality somewhere in their life—just not where they might expect it.

A holistic paradigm of sexual wellness includes a proclivity to explore our kinesphere (surrounding personal space), environment, and intimate relationships with curiosity and erotic, bodyful awareness. Sexual wellness is not about arriving at an ideal, performing and responding in a reliable and consistent manner. Instead, it is an awake relationship with the presence of desire and arousal with an awareness of how our early experiences and present social and relationship context may be impacting our experience of ourselves. It also incorporates an awareness that our desire and arousal can impact those around us, and we recognize that we have a personal responsibility within our relationships. This quality of awareness and navigation allows a trust and knowledge to develop within the self, trusting that we, to the best of our ability, challenge ourselves to be evermore awake and explore deeper levels of complexity.

Sexual Response Is So Much More Than You Think

In order to create an inclusive map of sexuality, we must dismantle the collective assumption that sex means a specific set of sexual behaviors (intercourse) or outcomes (orgasm) and take the laser focus off the genitals and sexual performance in order to view sex as a whole-person experience.

Often, we objectively look down at the body and make determinations about sexual performance—how hard, or wet, or exuberant we are. The original sexual response cycle, as developed through years of research by Masters and Johnson (1966), referred only to the physiological response of the body during sexual experience of consensual (we assume) intercourse. To be clear, they wanted to study something that had only been previously assumed: what exactly happens physiologically in the body during sex? They connected their participants (who were primarily white and reportedly heterosexual) to a myriad of data-gathering devices that measured things like heart rate, breathing, lubrication, and tumescence (engorgement of erectile tissue). According to the summation of Masters and Johnson's lab data, the cycle begins with excitement (physiological arousal of the body), continuing to plateau (increased excitement) just before orgasm (rhythmic contraction of the genitals accompanied by a release of tension and peak of pleasure), which is followed by resolution (a period of rest after orgasm) where the physiological arousal response subsides and the body returns to a resting state.

The human sexual response research was groundbreaking and became the basis for diagnosable sexual dysfunctions via sex therapist Helen Singer-Kaplan's triphasic model, which added desire as a prequel to sex and streamlined Masters and Johnson's work: desire, excitement, and orgasm, all with corresponding sexual disorder diagnoses (American Psychiatric Association, 2013).

The foundational models of Masters and Johnson and Kaplan gave sex therapists something tangible to leverage when helping their struggling and frustrated clients. Yet, introducing an overly efficient model like this to a misinformed and sex-fearful culture has had the unintended consequence of limiting healthy sexual experience to objective physiological responses. The sexual response cycle that was crafted from their data created a model that could apply to men and women. Therefore, not only does the model follow hetero-normative sexual function, to the exclusion of normal variability, it also does not consider the variability of genitals of different people or the impact of social and relational context on the internal experience of the sexual self. According to *Good Vibrations Guide to Sex* authors Winks and Semans: "Perhaps the only absolute truth about sexual response is how fundamentally fluid it is" (2002, pg. 30). In essence, human sexual responsiveness becomes limited in what is deemed "healthy" and excludes the experience of many sexually active people.

Although it has caused misunderstanding and rigidity around our cultural understanding of sex, the sexual response cycle can still be an applicable model with important modifications. Other models have surfaced since Masters and Johnson and Kaplan. The *Circular* model organizes the sexual response cycle into a circle, showing how satisfying sex feeds into desire for another sexual experience (Whipple & Brash-McGreer, 1997). Sex therapist Rosemary Basson's *Nonlinear* model recognizes the effect of emotional intimacy and relationship satisfaction (2001) on sexual responsiveness. Welcoming the sexual and reproductive organs as wise and inextricably interwoven systems of the body, while acknowledging the impact of the cultural and relational context, allows us to appreciate the healthy diversity of sexual responsiveness.

Like a wave building, cresting, and releasing, the underlying pattern of the sexual response cycle is found within all of us in both the magical and mundane moments of life. This rhythmic cycle is fundamental to how creative energy awakens, engages with the environment, and returns to us with new knowledge of ourselves that we can rest into and integrate.

Even those who identify as asexual—having no interest or desire for sex—have places in their lives where they experience this wave-like body rhythm. This sets the stage for the appreciation, acceptance, and cultivation of the sexual self in whatever form it takes. Sex educator and author Emily Nagoski (2015) also describes the experience of *arousal non-concordance*—when our heart or mind is turned on but our genitals are not, or when our genitals are aroused but the rest of is not interested in sexual contact. When the range of sexual response is expanded, when what being "turned on" feels like is opened up, the body can rest into acceptance of how one is showing up for the magic of connection. Instead of being the object of a laser-like judgmental focus, the genitals become an integral part of the whole self and are ready to express. Additionally, when we give ourselves space to learn how desire and arousal show up for us individually, we can make more informed decisions about the kind of sexual contact we may or may not want.

Now let's activate the experience-dependent mechanism of our nervous system and learn something new; let's *experience* sexual responsiveness as it is being discussed.

The Whole-Body Sexual Response

The human sexual response cycle is a brilliant engine of creativity. When we take the laser focus off the genitals and observe the qualities of sensation and movement throughout the *whole* body during sexual or sensual intimacy, we find a broader human experience. The way I see it, the stages in the cycle of sexual responsiveness (see Figure 5.1) are the very gears that fuel the overlapping waves of development and evolution in the human body. These components, through which we express our longing and our receptivity, are arranged in an elegant sequence to compel us to lean and reach toward what can fulfill us, inviting new experiences to incorporate into the home beneath our skin. After each cycle, we are different. After each cycle, we can integrate something new and become more of who we are. This is the value that I find when I explore with my clients how they embody this sequence in sex and in their creative endeavors. It is a tangible and readily available manifestation of generative energy, the energy that fuels our creativity and expression of purpose. This is not limited to just sexual activity but appears to support any creative endeavor, including dancing, giving birth, passion hobbies, eating—anyplace where aliveness is felt.

Remember the *Satisfaction Cycle* we discussed in Chapter 3? This is the developmental movement sequence presented by Bonnie Bainbridge-Cohen to describe how we engage with our enviornment for nourishment and learning. The Satisfaction Cycle, comprised of yield, push, reach, grasp, and pull, returning to yield, is a description of responsiveness and a call to exploratory movement. When it is woven into the human sexual response cycle, we gain an elegant template to explore how we embody the generative energy of the body in each moment. At each stage of the whole-person sexual response cycle, we can ask where Satisfaction Cycle was allowed to complete and where it was

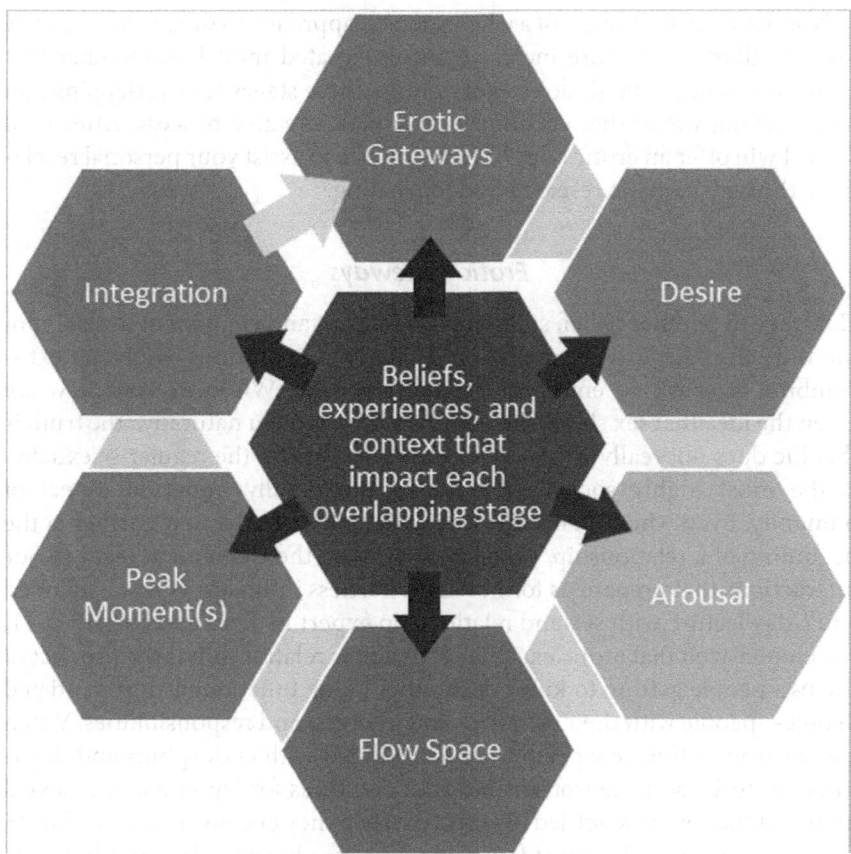

Figure 5.1   The Whole-Body Sexual Response Cycle

interrupted. As I explore how my clients embody the Satisfaction Cycle in the context of their sexual interests and behaviors, I keep in mind the words of somatic psychotherapist Arielle Schwartz: "the body does not just hold the memory of what happened to you, it holds the memory of what wanted to happen" (drarielleschwartz.com/somatic-therapy-in-trauma-treatment-dr-arielle-schwartz). What experiences of pleasure are we able to yield into? What desires were we able to reach for, grasp, and pull into ourselves? What pleasure experiences do we reach for but can't fully yield into because of a negative judgment that stands in our way? By following the sequence of movements of the Satisfaction Cycle at each stage of sexual response, we can access and reintegrate the full potential available to us. This opportunity does not happen with furtive or dissociated sex in the dark—true learning and evolution come from intentional and skillful engagement with the whole body.

Now let's visit each stage of a whole-person approach to the sexual response cycle to illustrate a more inclusive and integrated model. Remember that each stage is not a stand-alone experience—these stages are overlapping and interweaving waves that encompass a somatic creative process. After each stage, I will offer an erotic bodyfulness practice to assist your personal revelations through somatic research and journaling.

Erotic Gateways

Contrary to popular belief, spontaneous interest and enjoyment in sex is not the only normal. Environmental and personal conditions—our context—combine to spark an emergent arousal response. While we somehow are given the idea that sex should be "easy" or "just happen naturally," the truth is that life does not really set us up for erotic success on the regular—sexuality is the most highly socialized and environmentally impacted aspect of humanity. Even when we feel the magnetic pull toward a new partner at the beginning of a relationship, we take for granted the elements present in our interactions that prepare us for hot and effortless intimacy. When I attended a full-day lecture with sex and relationship expert Esther Perel back in 2011, she emphasized that erotic excitement in a new relationship is the product of the two people getting to know each other being functionally differentiated people—people with their own lives and interests and responsibilities. When we are around this new person, we are flooded with endorphins and dopamine (a "feel-good" neurotransmitter), conditions for "spontaneous" sexual arousal. Once we have settled in with a partner, they become more like family, and the exciting endorphin/dopamine response happens less and less. The exhilarating feeling of being in love settles into a more comfortable experience of love. Sex can begin to feel more like a chore or obligation.

A similar experience happens in how we relate to our lives. We settle into the trap of prioritizing responsibility and efficiency over the things that help us feel good and make our busy lives sustainable. We end up overscheduling the things that drain us instead of the things that replenish us. "Self-care" can feel like just another to-do on the list.

The unseen and often unappreciated elements that fill us up and allow us to access sensuality, pleasure, and excitement are the erotic gateways. Erotic gateways are the precursors to and activators of desire. Identifying and intentionally engaging erotic gateways help to define what supports active and intelligent engagement with the erotic body. By developing regular practices around the ways we prepare the earth of our bodies for intimacy, we can identify and own what our whole self needs to access desire and receptivity, whether we are engaging in restorative time off or are having solo or partnered sex. Erotic gateways become a discipline of self-care and personal resourcing. This can be quite empowering! We no longer need to rely on chance or our partner's efforts to be turned on—we can intentionally engage our erotic circuits to open to intimacy.

Erotic gateways are our entry into desire, the catalysts to a full-body pleasure experience—the contextual ground for eroticism. Containing the ingredients to unlock our erotic potential, these gateways meet the level of intensity in the body to open the senses to a place of yield—the state of receptivity to pleasure. These are the ways that we alleviate our everyday stress and anxiety, allowing us to be in the present moment with ourselves or our partner(s). The present moment is where we find our lived experience and the richness of what we desire.

Erotic gateways can be accessed through four overlapping areas of body awareness: physical (body movement, body experiences, experiencing music), mental (fantasy, choice, strategy), emotional (feelings, longings), and spiritual. Most often, people feel a combination of erotic gateways at play at the same time.

Physical: Physical erotic gateways are the things that activate the senses and physiology of the body directly through micro- or macro-movements. These are the activities that ease anxiety, stress, and frustration to bring the nervous system back into balance. A physical gateway can be highly active. After a long, stressful day at work, you hit the gym to exert your muscles to dissolve the stagnant tension by giving it direction. Now blood and oxygen are coursing through the body, releasing endorphins and activating the relaxation and pleasure response.

A physical gateway can also be more of a passive activity, such as receiving a massage or getting a good night of sleep from which we wake rested and relaxed and interested in connection. A physical erotic gateway is also listening to music or playing an instrument, feeling the vibrations of pleasurable sound penetrating our ears and our skin to pulsate our sensitive internal viscera. Physical gateways can also have an organizing quality like after cleaning and clearing a room in your house or finalizing a work project.

The fundamental principle here is whether you feel lighter, more aware, more relaxed, and curious than before you began the physical activity. This means that your nervous system has reached a place where stress has dissipated and the body is ready to be activated in a pleasurable way. Other physical erotic gateways include dance, adorning yourself for a night on the town, traveling to a vacation spot, or taking a bath.

Mental: Mental erotic gateways are accessed through the awareness of the mind. For example, what are your favorite fantasies? From a relaxing vision of lying on a beach to a fantasy with explicit sexual activity, intentionally conjuring up a mental vision can clear the mind of mundane stress and ignite desire and arousal. In the case of busy lovers or stretched-thin parents, a mental erotic gateway can be deciding on a time and place for intimacy. In this case, sex becomes a mental choice—"This afternoon will be a good time! Let's see if I can get my body on board." Prioritizing time for pleasure and closeness can be deeply meaningful and sexy, allowing arousal non-concordance to shift into an internally congruent experience of plea- sure. When we plan fun, sexy, or relaxing periods of time, we can access the magic of anticipation—that feeling of expectation that propels us forward in time. Other mental erotic gateways include the *eureka!* moment in problem- solving or participating in an engaging conversation.

Emotional: Emotional erotic gateways are rooted in an emotional desire for closeness or feeling an emotionally attuned connection. Because emo- tions happen in the body as energy-in-motion (e-motion), they are a direct gateway to work with body armor. In *Love Sense,* couples therapy expert Sue Johnson (2013) says, "Negative emotions, such as anger and fear, narrow our focus, while positive emotion expands the range of our thoughts and creates the urge to play and experiment" (pg. 81). These emotions can be engaged when we miss our partners due to distance from travel or work or during a connected moment with a partner when we feel the attunement from shar- ing love, grief, or celebration. In our relationship with ourselves, this can be a desire to connect with a feeling of love, compassion, or appreciation of ourselves. This emotional gateway can be surprising, so be on the lookout. I have seen clients connect with and validate themselves in their experience of anger or grief, only to peel away a barrier to feeling as a sudden warmth floods their body and a pleasurable surge of tingling emerges throughout their somatic landscape. Emotion as an erotic gateway is powerful and tran- scendent. This gateway could also be accessed again after peak moment(s), which you will see further into this chapter.

Spiritual: "In the transfiguration of the sensuous, the wildness of eros and the playfulness of the soul come into lyrical rhythm" (O'Donahue, 1998, pg. 31). A spiritual erotic gateway is an experience of connection, or a desire for connection, with that which is larger than ourselves. Or it is the awareness of a universal connection with humankind, with the divine, or with the flow of nature. This transpersonal gateway could look like sacred sexuality practices of circular breathing or eye-gazing, prayer, or the experience of transcen- dence during a physical/mental/emotional gateway moment. For others, this gateway could be connecting with nature during gardening or while on a hike. This is the gateway that, in the words of researcher Jenny Wade (2004), "shatters reality, opens new dimensions, rips the veil between the worlds, and produces ecstasies a thousand times more powerful than the most exquisite orgasm" (pg. 1).

It is important to note that what turns us on originally may be different from what leads us to the peak moment of sex. While cleaning the kitchen may be a physical and maybe mental erotic gateway, the act of washing coun- ters and stacking dishes probably won't bring you to orgasm (if it does, par- don my assumption). A gateway is a means of access or entry into a place which, while pleasurable in its own right, naturally opens to a further level of experience. For example, one person may like to begin with a soft massage (a physical erotic gateway) and gradually build in intensity while another person may want to begin with an intense spanking to drop out of the busy mind followed by slow, emotionally connected sex. Each individual has unique erotic gateways and progression to desire and arousal.

Erotic Bodyfulness Practice: Erotic Gateways

- *Journal practice: What are the erotic gateways that create within you a feeling of calmness and relaxation? What are the erotic gateways that create within you a feeling of excitement or anticipation?*
- *As you engage your erotic gateway, allow your attention to alternate between your thoughts (what you are thinking about or focusing on), your body (what parts of your body are sensorially alive and active), and your environment (what elements are present around you). Can you feel from the active places in your body what is around you (music, a dance partner, a conversation, etc.)? Now, with the help of your breath, invite your body to reach out and connect with your environment. Notice the impact on your feeling self.*

Desire

Desire is a result of accessing the erotic gateways and is expressed as a leaning toward connection, union, and pleasure. Desire is longing, the unarguable tug toward a source of arousal. While arousal is the heat and sensation of the erotic, desire gives arousal *direction*. Like a wise inner compass, desire directs you to your growing edges and your next level of erotic evolution. In her Nonlinear model of sexual response, clinical professor Rosemary Basson (2005) identifies two types of sexual desire: spontaneous and responsive. Spontaneous desire is desire for sexual contact, which seems to happen automatically with little stimulation, while responsive desire is a want for sexual contact that builds over time with pleasurable touch, emotional connection, or engagement with a pleasurable activity that shifts body physiology into a receptive state. Based on her research, the difference between these two types of desire are most often connected to gender—cisgender men are more likely to experience spontaneous desire, while cisgender women are more likely to experience responsive desire. However, in my counseling experience, this gender divide is far too simplistic and not representative of many of the clients that I see. These two types of desire are also connected to length and type of relationship—cisgender women tend to experience more spontaneous desire while dating or at the beginning of a relationship and transition into responsive desire after a period of time with one partner. Again, there is much variability beyond Basson's research conditions.

Desire is not just a physical desire for sexual contact; it can also be of an emotional nature. You may notice that you have an interest in skin-to-skin contact with a partner when you miss them, feel emotionally or mentally connected with them, or want to begin the day feeling connected. Even though you may not be sexually excited, the emotional form of desire is also normal and valid.

When we focus our attention to our interoceptive senses in desire, the internal sensations and movement impulses, we find that we are internally leaning toward a lover even before we physically extend our arms to reach for them and pull them closer to us. When we focus our attention on an even finer level, we may find that we are already pulling them toward us, taking them in with our eyes, our skin, and our breath. When I work with a couple in my office, I encourage my clients to extend their senses to feel their partner before they even touch—to learn about how they are already enveloping them with their senses.

Repulsion, the opposite of desire, directs us away from a source of arousal. As in physics, a repulsive force is the force that causes particles or bodies to repel one another. When we allow the interoceptive senses of the body to tell us what the source of the repulsion is, we can learn about and better articulate what we are saying "no" to in the moment. Desire can be present throughout a sexual experience, ebbing and flowing, rising and falling for the duration and beyond. While erotic gateways are the red carpet up to the door, desire is the force that seduces us over the threshold again and again. Desire keeps our attention and body transfixed throughout an experience of sexual pleasure. Even though desire is represented in Figure 5.1 as one area of the whole-body sexual response cycle, desire keeps us turning toward pleasure and intimacy—it is the "yes" to arousal, "yes" to the flow space, "yes" to the peak moments, "yes" to integration, and "yes" to doing it all again. Desire is the "yes" that invites us back into connection after disconnection.

Erotic Bodyfulness Practice: Dedicated to Desire

- *What do you desire in sex? What keeps you transfixed and moving toward pleasure? What are the activities and quality of connection that inspires your arousal to build, to spread to other areas of your body, to reignite after a sexual encounter?*
- *When you are in the presence of something that you desire, take a few full breaths in and full breaths out with the core of your*

> *body—expanding rib cage, belly, and pelvis. Can you perceive in your muscles an opening and softening in the direction of what you desire? Can you perceive any other sensations accompanying the opening? Perhaps tingling or bubbling in your belly or throat? Draw a basic body map and, like a topographical map of a landscape, color the corresponding areas of your body with shapes and textures to represent the sensations you notice.*
>
> • *What causes your desire to wane or turn you off? Notice the quality of your breath now. Can you perceive a tightening or constriction on your muscles, causing you to lean away from the source of repulsion?*

Arousal

Arousal is your lived experience of being turned on, turned off, or some combination of the two. Arousal ignites a complex lived experience of full-body muscle tension, relaxation, and flow of fluids and hormones found in the body. It is also marked by a quickened heartbeat and increased blood flow to the whole body, which activates the erectile response in all types of genitals. Everyone has a similar amount of erectile tissue.

Pleasurable arousal has the potential to be an anchor and an internal resource. When aroused, the mother-tongue language of the body can inform the whole self on what to move toward to savor, to experience satisfaction, and to expand personal growth potential. By paying close attention to the bodily experience of arousal, and identifying what ignites it in the environment, we can begin to relate with the location of our growing edges.

There are as many ways that arousal lives in the body as there are people; while there is much overlap between us, your full-bodied arousal landscape is unique to you. The way that your body holds and circulates the sensation of arousal is determined by the patterns of muscle tension and range of movement in body. At the extremes, arousal can be the slow lava flow meeting the ocean, hardening and cooling the creative fire. Arousal can also feel like the spark whipped up by a sudden gust of wind, overtaking the landscape of the body and emotions too quickly to manage.

When bound- and free-flow muscle tensions are engaged with intention and malleability, it is like expertly surfing a wave. Remember from Chapter 3 that bound-flow and *fighting attributes* are present with high-energy excitement, cautious feelings or boundary-setting behavior, while free-flow and *indulging attributes* are present with more carefree feelings and a yielding into experience. When I invite clients to explore their relationship to arousal, I invite them to witness their internal environment and notice when free-flow (indulging) and bound-flow (fighting/learning) qualities arise.

When arousal has more of a free-flow quality to it, there can be a simultaneous relaxation and a spreading sense of excitement, warmth, tingling, and pleasure in large areas of the body. Indulgent qualities open us to a heightened experience of pleasure, satisfaction, and even multiple orgasms. An overflow of free-flow or indulging rhythms can also lead to difficulty in discerning when and where we express our arousal—we need some bound flow to help us modulate expression. Too much free flow can feel like being out of control and groundless. These are the moments when one can have a difficult time discerning personal boundaries, touch others without consent, or bump into others with a seeming lack of awareness of the space around them. Too much free flow of arousal energy can also cause one to dissociate from their body—we all have an "upper limit" to the amount of arousal we can tolerate in any given time before we disconnect from sensation and awareness.

When arousal has a bound or fighting quality to it, one can feel sensation and expression narrowed. Like a bottleneck in a canyon, flow is constricted and increasingly dense in nature. Bound-flow arousal is characterized by more localized pleasure of the body, shallow and fast breath, a sensation of anxiety, discomfort, or feeling anticipatory or rushed. Too much bound-flow arousal leads to dissatisfaction, a feeling of emptiness, a lack of sensation, or a tension that cannot be relieved. It can also lead to an unconscious expression of arousal, missing or disregarding the consent of another, and a localized flash-paper pleasure that disappears almost as quickly as it ignited. When bound flow is more prominent than free flow, we are denied the full-body pleasure waves that are available.

To be clear, both bound- and free-flow rhythms are needed in arousal—the free flow allows for the relaxation and movement necessary for heightened sensation and yielding into pleasure, while bound flow is necessary to excite and activate peak moments like orgasm. An overflow of either indulgent or fighting rhythms can obstruct awareness of self and our impact on others. When the indulgent and fighting rhythms of arousal are in active balance and feel enjoyable, we refer to the somatic experience of being "turned on"—a simultaneous relaxation and excitation in the nervous system, heat, quickened breath, and a captivated focus. As we progress in sexual complexity, we become awake to what enlivens us and what inhibits us—what activates indulging qualities or fighting qualities. When we are able to oscillate between free and bound flow in arousal, we feel balanced and discerning as tension builds and releases.

This bound- and free-flow oscillation of sexual energy is mirrored in the dual-control model of sex educator and researcher Emily Nagoski (2015). She describes the process of an individual learning how to hit their accelerators to turn on the "ons" (free-effort flow sexual energy) and learning what pushes the brakes to turn off your "offs" (bound-effort flow sexual energy). It is common to experience complex arousal in intimate experiences in which we feel both pleasure and discomfort, either at the same time or in alternating waves. Both the brakes and accelerators are active. Intimate touch, closeness, and skin-to-skin contact can be pleasurable, exciting, and emotionally regulating. Intimate contact can also evoke self-consciousness, anxiousness, or a freeze response due to negative messages or experiences related to intimacy or sexuality. This variability is normal.

When exploring arousal during intimacy, invite awareness through what somatic sex therapist Stella Resnick calls in *Body-to-Body Intimacy* (2018) the *erotoceptive senses*, the seventh sense found in the erogenous zones of the body. Erogenous zones contain some of the most tightly packed nerves of our whole body. These sensory neurons are charged with the purpose of acutely sensing how the environment impacts the most tender parts of the body. When we turn our attention away from the self-conscious mind and begin to "think" from our erotoceptive senses, the intimate experience becomes pleasurably immersive.

As we activate the erotoceptive senses, we also engage with kinesthetic senses, the sensory neurons that allow for awareness of body position and movement. When we are aroused, body movement begins to shift from everyday navigation to a sequencing of movement in response to the direction given by desire—the body organizes itself to move closer to the desired experience. When we simultaneously move with and are moved by our kinesthetic senses, our body rhythms have arrived at the flow space of sexual response—where free-flow and bound-flow muscle tension are balanced for an effortless quality of pressing into the points of pleasure and yielding into the sensation.

Learning to dance with arousal through your bound- and free-flow muscle tension qualities is an important part of the somatic creative process.

Erotic Bodyfulness Practice: Awakening Arousal

- *Activate bodyful awareness to learn your tension-flow somatic map.*
- *Begin by visualizing or performing a pleasurable and non-overtly sexual activity like dancing, making art, or eating something delicious.*
  - *As you engage in this activity, activate awareness from your facial muscles, chest area, solar plexus (diaphragm area), belly, and pelvis one area at a time. Take your time in each area of your body to notice the quality of muscle tension and sensation found in each. Remember to be as descriptive as possible.*
- *Choose a sexy visualization or image or experience that activates pleasurable arousal for you.*

> - *As you begin to experience the arousal energy, activate awareness from your facial muscles, chest area, solar plexus (diaphragm area), belly, and pelvis one area at a time. Take your time in each area of your body to notice the quality of muscle tension and sensation found in each. Again, take the time to describe in detail.*
>
> - *As you learn how the bound-flow and free-flow muscle tension show up in your body, explore how breath, posture adjustment, and movement help you to access both. Through free-flow arousal, learn how your breath and movement allow pleasure and sensation to circulate through your whole body, how you can soften and yield into pleasure, and flow with a sexual partner from one intimate moment to the next without hesitation or abruptness. Through bound-flow arousal, learn how your breath and movement help you slow down, change activities, and set boundaries or stop yourself when a partner sets a boundary.*

Flow Space

In the whole-person sexual response cycle, flow space replaces Masters and Johnson's *plateau* stage. Beyond the buildup of sensation toward orgasm, flow space is the moment when the dance between bound- and free-flow muscle tension finds balance in the body. As arousal builds in the body and the contraction and relaxation of your muscles flow, one into the other, there is a sense of moving and being moved simultaneously. As Csikszentmihalyi (2014) said about the creative state of *flow*, when we are aroused at this level, we can do our best learning. When we reach the flow space of arousal, we are at the peak place of learning, as we have access to a vast range of pleasurable sensation.

When we activate erotic bodyfulness practice within the flow space, a whole universe of insights and expansion of our learning edge is realized. The learning edge is the border between what is known and what is not yet known, and on this edge of knowing is our next level of realized personal potential. A writer could experience this moment as their fingers type the words just fast enough to keep up with the words flowing from their mind. Or the dancer who is so engrossed in the movement of their body that they lose a sense of time and are unaware of the exhaustion building in their muscles as they express more fully than ever before. This is what we identify as *passion*. In passionate moments, we do things we never thought possible.

Most often, the flow space is quickly exited through orgasm with a frenetic pace that charges toward an endpoint that lands flat. The invitation here is to slow down and savor this effortless and delicious space. Flow space may come and go multiple times during a creative activity or a sexual experience, so allow it to ebb and flow without trying to grasp onto it. Once you grasp, it will slip through your fingers. While in the flow space, expand just a little further, breathe just a little deeper to help keep the experience afloat.

Erotic Bodyfulness Practice: Flow Space

- *Engage in a pleasurable activity that you experience some mastery with. As you engage in this activity, practice erotic bodyfulness. Oscillate between the awareness of the activity and the somatic landscape of your body. At the moments when you feel the effortless quality of performing the activity, you may feel a lightness, a soft surge of pleasure. Now, breathe into every cell in the body at once. Expand the pleasure into your pelvis and reach out from the core of your body through your body endpoints of hands, feet, pelvic floor, and top of your head. Soften your body and your focus. Allow your torso to reach up through your shoulders and out your palms and fingertips, engage in-breath and awareness to invite the sensation in your pelvis to reach down through your legs and out your toes, and expand your spine through your tailbone and out through the crown of your head. These movements could be micro-movements or large movements and are directed by your in-breath and yielded into with your out-breath. Like a winged creature lifted up by the breeze, let your body almost hang in the air, your in-breath lifting you as your out-breath softens you. This experience is like floating your body in water as your breath works with the buoyancy of the water to keep you above the surface.*

Peak Moments

Peak moments can be a genital orgasm, an intense emotional moment, or the "aha!" moment of the scientist. These are the moments that pleasurable, bound energy has been reintroduced to the flow space, heightening the nervous system into a crescendo of pleasure and emotion. It can even activate the reflex of orgasm. The more senses that are awake and aware, the more power and growth is born from the experience. In *Urban Tantra* (2007), author Barbara Carrellas offers many alternatives to the genital orgasm. A *mindgasm* happens when we solve a mental problem or discover a mind-blowing idea. We experience a *heartgasm* when we have an intense emotional experience or connection. And a *bodygasm* can happen while dancing, painting, or even giving birth. In other words: peak moments are a multifaceted and multi-contextual euphoric experience.

Peak moments are marked by a dramatic release of endorphins, oxytocin, and other feel-good internal chemicals and hormones—the tip of an altered-state iceberg. Arriving at peak moments requires a solid buildup time and just enough risk balanced with safety to surrender to the experience. In BDSM (bondage, domination/discipline, submission/sadism, masochism) and kink play, the peak moment is also described as *sub-space* (the euphoric state of the submissive partner) or *dom-space* (the euphoric state of the dominant partner), an experience of euphoria, vastly heightened sensation, or a transcendent out-of-body experience. In her research, sex therapist Dulcinea Pitagora (2017) describes this state as "characterized by activation of the sympathetic nervous system, the release of epinephrine and endorphins, and a subsequent period of nonverbal, deep relaxation. This altered state of consciousness may include temporary feelings of depersonalization and derealization" (pg. 46).

Erotic Bodyfulness Practice: Peak Moment

Begin this practice with a nonsexual, pleasurable activity like dancing, running, painting, doing martial arts, watching a favorite movie, or listening to music. After you decide on your activity, notice your anticipation preceding it and the experience of your body as you begin the activity. Oscillate your whole-body awareness from what your senses detect (taste, sight, touch, sound, kinesthetic) and their impact on your somatic landscape as you engage in the activity. Back and forth, in-breath and out-breath, allowing your breath to pool around the areas of heightened sensory experience. Notice the moments where you feel a flow state—that active yet effortless buoyancy between your activity and your somatic experience of the activity. Now, can you identify a moment or moments when you felt an intense moment of pleasure? Perhaps you experienced an emotional release, a "runner's high" while running or dancing, a "eureka" moment while painting, the moment of revelation in the movie where the mystery is solved and all the disparate pieces fall into place. Describe your somatic landscape and movement impulses that ignite in these peak moments.

Now explore during a solo or partner sex experience. Can you identify a moment or moments during the sexual encounter where you felt an emotional peak, pleasurable rhythmic contractions of your arousal anatomy, a full-body surge of lightness and electricity, or a beautiful, dream-like vision? These are all peak moments. Make note of how it is expressed within you. What are the similarities and what are the differences between nonsexual and sexual peaks?

Integration

Instead of the resolution phase in the Masters and Johnson sexual response cycle, integration is the period after the peak moment(s) when our bodies access a place of deep relaxation. This is a time for "pillow talk," restorative movements or stillness, or a review of what was enjoyed and learned during the experience. This is such an important period of time. Beyond the rest and relaxation at this stage, integration is the space where you can appreciate the learning experience and savor the opportunity to connect, even if the erotic experience didn't go the way you thought or expected. Whether the experience was solo or with a partner, sharing gratitude and practicing erotic bodyfulness can support a positive relationship and lay the ground for positive erotic moments in the future.

In the integration phase after a partnered erotic experience, some people may want to take a moment to themselves to visit the bathroom, get a drink, and connect with themselves. Others may want to stay close with a partner. This depends on your attachment style and relational dynamic. Having a different way of approaching integration can cause hurt feelings, misunderstandings, or conflict for partners. Couples therapist and author Stan Tatkin (2012) talks about the different attachment styles and their respective ways of processing experiences and emotions. Some people are more *wave*-like, emotionally leaning into a partner for connection, reassurance, and relational processing of experiences. *Island*-like people, however, process experiences and emotions more internally and separately from their partners. When we understand that our partner may simply have a different style of integration, we are less likely to take this personally. This is tricky because erotic experiences uncover our most vulnerable selves, so talking about your integration style with your partner can be helpful by creating what Tatkin calls the *couple-bubble*, in which partners help each other get what they need without compromising themselves.

Erotic Bodyfulness Practice: Integration

After a pleasurable nonsexual experience or a sexual experience with yourself or a partner, how do you generally transition out from the intensity of the erotic environment? Do you notice that you have the impulse to shift quickly? Do you engage in another activity, rush to the bathroom, get dressed, or go to sleep directly after? Do you notice that you have the impulse to linger? Do you enjoy talking about the experience, cuddling with a partner while sharing your thoughts and feelings, or journaling? Do you find that you want something similar or different than your partner? Can you find a way to satisfy both sets of needs?

> *Try incorporating some sort of integration practice after an erotic experience, such as journaling about your solo sex time, bathing yourself lovingly, sharing with a partner what you enjoyed about the experience or about them, what you noticed about your own sexual evolution, or maybe a vision you had during a peak moment. During and afterward, see how your chosen integration practice feels in your somatic landscape.*

The Embedded Center and Surrounding Context

In the center of this sequence (see Figure 5.1) is the internal landscape of our body where beliefs, values, sense of identity, and body memories reside. These elements that we have integrated within ourselves from our experiences can positively or negatively impact us in each stage of the sexual sequence. Embedded deep within the nervous system of us all are our personal experiences of our family and sociocultural location. As mentioned previously, our nervous system is experience dependent, so the experiences that we have related to our body, sexuality, and relationships influence what and how we respond thereafter. When it comes to negative experiences, we unfortunately cannot simply say, "Oh, that was in the past." The reality is that all our experiences live within us in every moment. Like a bonsai tree consistently pruned over the years, our experiences influence the direction and shape that we take. Our sexual response sequence is influenced by our experiences around touch and the messages received about the body and sexuality. We may have a secure and fulfilling relationship with the sexual self or we may feel confusion, discomfort, or a distortion related to sexuality. More than likely, you may find that you have a bit of both—there are aspects of your sexuality in which you feel confident and fulfilled while other areas activate discomfort and dysregulation.

When we find ourselves in an uncomfortable body position, upset by the memory of a disturbing experience during sex, or find that the body is tightening against opening to arousal, this is an opportunity to slow down. Instead of pushing through the discomfort, back up to the moment in the erotic experience when you felt safe enough and interested in opening to pleasure. Give yourself permission to slow down and acknowledge that your body is communicating something important: that it wants and needs something different or that your body wants to repair the impact of a prior difficult experience. Emphasize your out-breath, be held by your partner, or allow your body to do some physical shaking (like a rag doll) to work the stuck energy through a movement sequence. Listen *from* your body for guidance about what it needs and breathe gratitude into your body for communicating to you what is needed. A powerful healing moment is missed when we push or rush past these important stuck moments.

Somatic teacher and lecturer Staci Haines (2007) says that as you increase your ability to feel sensations in the body, you can better detect the subtleties of your emotions. Haines points out the importance of this in the healing process: "when we are able to feel the depths of these emotions, we experience transformation and release. That metamorphosis and return to empowerment is what we mean by *healing*" (pg. 175). The more you are fluent in the language of the body, the more powerful your healing potential.

Erotic Bodyfulness Moment: The Embedded Center

- *At what stage in the above illustrated sexual response cycle do you find that you get stuck, shut down, become uncomfortable, or rush through?*
- *If you find that you have trouble accessing erotic gateways, what are the ways you can shore up your skills to self-resource, participate in things that you enjoy, and set personal and professional boundaries that make more room for you and what is important to you?*
- *Do you notice difficulty accessing desire, the impulse of arousal energy to move in a direction? What is your relationship to desire? Do you feel that you have social or community support for who or what you desire? Are you allowed to experience desire or is this an experience that feels unattainable?*
- *How does arousal live in your body? This is the sensory experience underlying the entirety of the sexual response. When you begin to experience arousal, do you notice memories or feelings surface that feel familiar? Can you move your arousal energy with your breath, or does this feel challenging? What is the sensation of the obstacle to moving your arousal energy?*
- *When you arrive in the flow space of a sexual experience, do you find that you can stay in active engagement? What is your pacing or speed? Do you feel an urgency to get to the next state of peak moment or orgasm? This is often the place where my clients report experiences such as having a sense of anxiety about maintaining erection, get distracted, experience a rising fear of their inability to have an orgasm or orgasming "too quickly," or fear of a sexual partner getting bored. From where do these fears and anxieties originate?*
- *What is your relationship to the peak moment(s)? Do you find that you have an effortless relationship with genital orgasm? Do you find*

> *that you get stuck in flow space and give up on rising to any peak?*
> *Do you experience a peak moment and then feel a rising discomfort*
> *in your body?*
> * *When the time for integration arrives, do you find that you have an*
>   *intense desire to stay close to a sexual partner? Do you experience*
>   *repulsion and a need to quickly separate? Are you able to verbalize*
>   *what you enjoyed or appreciate your partner or do you find that you*
>   *drop into criticism of yourself or a partner?*

Transitions: More Than Getting From Place to Place

We live in a hurried culture, rushing from one project to the next or one place to the next. In sex, we freight-train through "foreplay" to get the "main event," usually intercourse or orgasm. Rushing through the moments and phases of sex gets us quickly past any shadows or shame that we are harboring—old sexual-schema triggers that we unconsciously replay to our insistent dissatisfaction. These are the automatic and assumed scenarios that we graft together from our sociocultural sources and experiences, which play themselves out like a puppeteer controlling a marionette.

These often unconscious and un-scrutinized sexual stories keep us limited and prevent us from making more awake, more satisfying sexual choices. They also bar us from truly savoring the pleasure and self-knowledge to be found in the moments of transition. They hinder embodied consent. In short, rushing through sex keeps us from getting the sex that we truly, deeply want.

So, let's slow this down. Between each stage of the whole-person sexual response cycle is a transition, a tension, and a release. Transitions are not just blinks of the eyes between big events—these bridges are significant moments to savor and to study. Each moment is a gateway into the next. As we slow down our awareness of time, we gain access to unconscious beliefs, movement impulses, emotional expressions, and the truth of our consent to sexual engagement. It is in these in-between spaces that we forge new, more inclusive and fulfilling experiences and sexual schemas. It is in the transition, in the realm of potent stillness between in-breath and out-breath, in the lengths of fascia that connect the large muscles of the body, that each new impulse for movement is born and detected. Between desire and arousal, there are innumerable awakenings of sensation and connection. Between flow space and peak moments is the buildup followed by the gratifying, cascading chaos of release. Between peak moments and integration, our old templates of attachment are initiated. Therefore, it is in the same transitional spaces that the power to rewrite templates, to make a different turn at each crossroad, is found.

Diving Deeper Into Arousal: Enjoyment and Responsibility

Having an awake and intelligent relationship with arousal is the single most important skill that we can develop as sexual beings. When we are asleep in our arousal—taking it for granted, believing our arousal trajectory is more important than someone else's comfort, or simply not paying attention—we can experience everything from dissatisfaction to outright harm. Developing responsibility over our own arousal and not taking responsibility for the arousal of others is a revolutionary thing. To begin this awake-arousal journey is to develop a core relationship skill and true sovereignty in relationship to our own body.

Just as it is not sensible to pitch ourselves headlong and un-resourced into an uncharted forest, it is important that we learn to navigate arousal with open eyes and with discipline. We pack our backpack with food, water, extra clothing, a compass, and flashlights (with extra batteries) to be resourced and prepared for the journey. When navigating the territory of arousal, we bring with us the bodyful skills of breath, movement, multimodal awareness, and trust in the language of the body. We may even bring along a willing partner or hire a guide, a sex therapist or sex educator trained to give others the tools to cultivate intelligent eroticism. To truly understand our experience of arousal, we must also consider the environment in which our erotic bodies have awoken and matured and practice the skills of embodied arousal. Like Westley and Buttercup in the Fire Swamp in *The Princess Bride*, we can learn to anticipate our individual obstacles and overcome the challenges we face from within ourselves and within the sociocultural environment in which we live and work and love.

When we are in an aroused state and untrained in somatic navigation, the inhibitory part of our brain turns off and we are more likely to act from our unconscious selves. This can invoke the feeling of being out of control, of saying "yes" when part of us wanted to say "no," or of missing or misreading the cues of a sexual partner. When intelligent eroticism is online, we can master the dance of arousal expression and containment, like a surfer deftly riding an ocean wave. We intentionally engage movement and breath to make moment-to-moment micro-adjustments, responding to the interplay between our somatic landscape and the external erotic environment. In essence, we can train to become more awake and more skillful while in a state of sexual arousal. This is an important element of the somatic creative process.

To refine the radical skill of embodied arousal, I present my clients with a simple (yet so complex!) map. The concentric model of arousal emphasizes awareness and enjoyment of somatic experience, identification of social and cultural influences, and ownership over our expression (Figure 5.2). It encourages developing skills to circulate arousal within the body in order

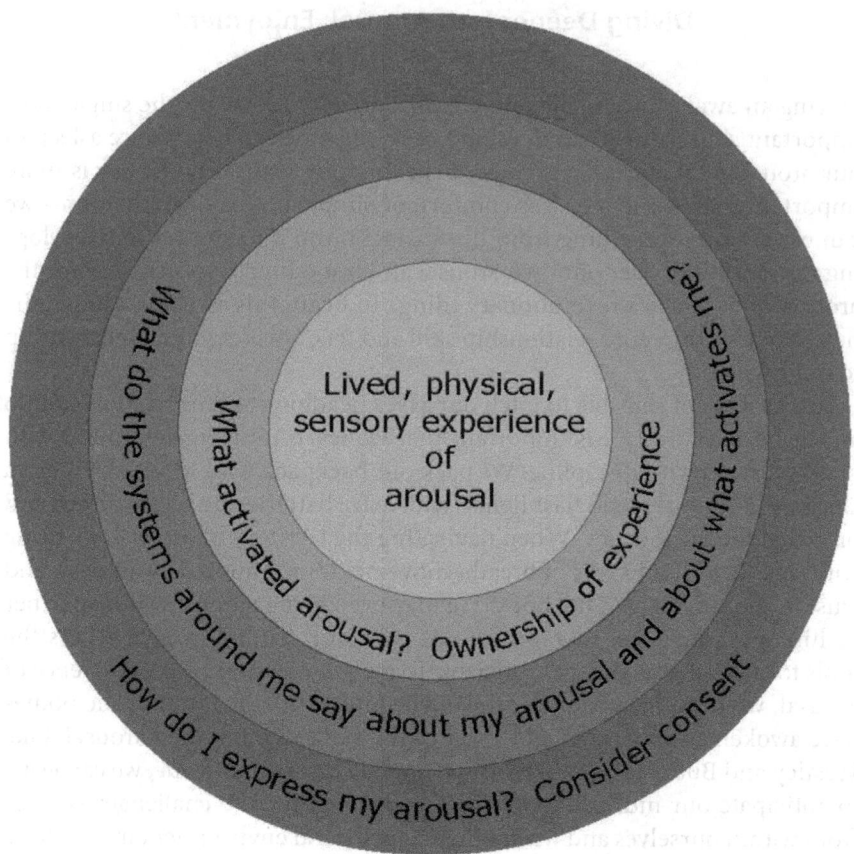

Figure 5.2 Concentric Model of Arousal by Melissa Walker, MA, LPC, CST, R-DMT

to channel it where we choose in a responsive and consensual way versus a reactive or out-of-control way.

When I share this model with clients, I invite them to first visualize something or someone that turns them on, something that ignites an experience of sexual arousal in the body. You can do this now so that you have something to work with as we travel through the concentric circles. Once the image is vivid in your mind or sitting right in front of you in the form of a physical image or person, you can begin to visit each layer of the map.

In the center of this map is the somatic landscape of the body. This is the inner field where arousal emerges and makes its mark. As sexual arousal or turn-on awakens in your body, take an inventory of your internal experience. Temperature. Bound- or free-flow muscle tension. Rate of heartbeat. Location of breath. Movements or gestures. Combining these somatic aspects creates a map of how arousal can show up within you.

The second layer investigates what your arousal is attributed to. Not simply about who or what turns you on—at this level, we are looking at the qualities and attributes of the inspiration for your turn-on. If this is a person, what are their personality characteristics? The way they move, the way they look at you? If your arousal is attributed to an activity, what are the qualities of the activity? Who is with you, where are you, what is the nature of the elements of an activity? Make note of the qualities, as if recording the whole important elements of a dream. What activates arousal within us, excites our senses and draws us in, are the qualities that exist at our growing edge. For example, perhaps we hold a lot of bound flow in our body and we see someone who has mastered a flow and freedom of movement. As you explore what has ignited your arousal, what do you notice happens to your somatic landscape? Is the map of sensation the same or different? Heightened, perhaps? Remember, the more deeply and vividly we explore the pertinent elements, the more arousal may surge from within.

The third layer is an opportunity to look at how your sociocultural environment impacts your arousal. When you visualize yourself enjoying your arousal response with your visualization, how do you think your family, religion, community, or larger culture would react to you upon learning that this is what turns you on? This process identifies the social influences that we have internalized—the verbal and nonverbal messages that impact our expression even without our conscious awareness. This is what we call *introjection* in the world of psychotherapy—the unconscious adoption of the attitudes or beliefs of others. Oscillate back into the center circle, your inner landscape, and notice what happens to your somatic map as you imagine yourself being witnessed. Is your somatosensory experience the same now or is it different? Do you feel more free flow or bound flow in your body? What shows up here can be a positive influence, allowing more free-flow energy in your body and a feeling of self-affirmation. Or it can invoke a negative response, increasing the bound-flow muscle tension and an experience of feeling bad about the self. The fundamental question, once you become aware of your social ecology, is whether you can let yourself enjoy your arousal and therefore enjoy being in your body. The answer to this is complex and helps to identify where in your social life you feel supported and where you feel you must inhibit your sexuality.

The final layer of this map investigates how you channel your arousal based on the experience of the preceding layers. When you experience arousal in response to that person across the room and you believe that your family would view you in a negative or positive light, how do you express your turn-on? Again, oscillate back into the centermost circle of your internal somatic landscape and notice your impulse for movement. Are you now standing with arms wide open and with full breath? Or are you twisting and turning away with bound-flow muscle tension? How you are now inhabiting your body is how you relate to your sexual arousal.

You now have a model to explore and understand more about your embodied experience of arousal. With this newfound awareness let's turn to the relationship between arousal and consent.

Informed and Embodied Consent

Sexual arousal has been described over the centuries as being chained to an out-of-control lunatic or madman. When we do not tend to the knowledge of our own body or consent, this can be disastrous. But it does not have to be this way. When consent is actively being tended, arousal can lead us to a transcendent realm. Practicing erotic bodyfulness during partner sex gives us tools to know what we are saying "yes" to, what we are saying "no" to, and where we need to slow down to assess our level and direction of interest. When we better understand what ignites our arousal and how arousal feels in our body, we increase our sexual and relational intelligence and we make smarter choices about when to express and when to contain. This is the bedrock of embodied consent and personal responsibility. In an age where consent as a core component of sexual dialogue is finally taking a front seat in our culture, having the skills to verbally and nonverbally navigate sexual situations is a hot commodity.

The trouble is that arousal can make communication difficult. Whether to request a desire or set a boundary, sex education and sociocultural messages about sexuality do not prepare us well to develop the skill of present-moment awareness while aroused. In her masters paper on embodied consent, somatic psychotherapist Emma Daley identifies the challenge this presents in a thought-centric culture: "Consent has traditionally been represented as an act of the mind, an agreement that absolves parties of potentially violative behavior" (2020, pg. 10).

When we learn about sex in anxiety-provoking environments, our ability to articulate our desire verbally is diminished. Our fight-flight-freeze response is activated and we take a protective stance, inhibiting the ability of verbal communication. We may not be able to verbally speak during sex at all! This is why we cannot simply rely on our verbal ability to communicate consent. Daley goes on to say that "words are far more useful for talking about past, future, and anything else that only exists conceptually. Nonverbal cues are better at communicating feeling states and emotional intentions" (pg. 15). Therefore, we must cultivate a curious and welcoming space to learn how we and our partners express sexual consent and dissent nonverbally, while also encouraging but not expecting verbal communication. The more awake our relationship while in the altered state of arousal, the more communication of desire and boundaries is possible.

Developing an intimate relationship with your own arousal is an empowering and growth-oriented activity. Explore sensory play and notice what initiates a pleasurable response from the body. Begin with what feels interesting to you and stay with it until your body "asks" for something else or something more. The "ask" for more can feel like an opening and "leaning toward" in the body. Take time to learn how your body seeks out and responds to pleasure. You may find that your body expresses arousal response through warmth, a throbbing or aching, tingling, a "reaching" from deep within muscles, or a leaning toward or softening with contact. See the erotic bodyfulness practice in Chapter 4 for guided practice. Remember that a lack of arousal is not commentary on your gender-role status or the functioning of your body—rather, it is an inner hand pointing your attention to something important. This is an invitation to explore the presenting body armor and what it is trying to keep safe. Thank your body for giving you important information to keep you safe and return to the present moment for further exploration. This is information that you can then share with a sexual partner prior to intimacy or keep in mind for yourself to communicate a slowing down or pause during intimacy.

Your body needs a balance between safety and novelty to activate and stay awake to sexual arousal. This balance looks different for everyone. Safer partner sex may include open communication, an emotional connection, accurate knowledge of arousal anatomy, sex toys and sensory objects, or the sharing of preferences and boundaries. Ask yourself what allows you to feel safer and communicate this to a sexual partner prior to sex. When you include novelty in partner sex, from massage style contact and kissing, to paddles and piercing (and beyond), talk with your sexual partner about nonverbal signs that you may be too activated to communicate in a direct or obvious way. You may find that your eyes widen without blinking, your breath gets tight, or your body becomes more rigid. Sharing this information with a partner increases the likelihood of a positive sexual experience.

Of course, studying your own arousal also requires a look at the substances that you may use. When alcohol, cannabis, or other substances are present in the body, this can open the body too wide by forcibly reducing inhibition. I recommend to my clients that they create a sober space to work on embodied consent in the beginning. After that, if they choose to have a glass of wine prior to sex, practice a mindful drinking practice. Take time to closely monitor how the substance that you choose impacts your somatic arousal map, how it affects your ability to use your voice to indicate consent, and how it impacts your connection with a sexual partner.

Integrating an Inclusive Map of Sexual Response

You now have a new lens to view the somatic landscape of sexual energy in your body. Beyond the functioning of your sexual organs, your sexual responsiveness is a whole-body dance between bound- and free-flow energy, a push-reach-grasp-pull-yield sequence of connection with pleasure and creative growth. You have been given the option to explore the cultivation of your sexuality through both sexual and nonsexual pathways. Along the way, you may have discovered aspects of your sexual response that feel exciting and integrated. You may have also discovered aspects of your sexual response that feel blocked in an incomplete satisfaction cycle. This is all okay. In the following chapters, you will be given the opportunity to learn more about the erotic obstacles and be given more somatic tools to open the gates for a full-bodied expression of your sexuality.

6

THE EMBEDDED SEXUAL SELF

There is a tapestry woven in the dance between the felt experience of our sexuality and intimacy with others. This tapestry, woven from our experience in a social body, influences our felt sense, our engagement with others, and the experience others have of us. In *The Good Vibrations Guide to Sex*, sex experts Winks and Semans (2002) underscore the importance of recognizing "the huge influence that subjective conditions, social factors, and psychological readiness have on our experience of sex" (pg. 30). As we dive into the deeper layers of the somatic sexual self, it is time to consider the central ways in which upbringing, relationships, and the intersection of your social locations (your gender, race, ethnicity, age, body and cognitive ability, class, relationship status, body size, etc.) impact the ways you inhabit your body.

Embodiment is a state of inter-corporeality, emphasizing that "the experience of being embodied is never a private affair, but is always already mediated by our continual interactions with other human and nonhuman bodies" (Weiss, 1998, pg. 5). This underlying principle acknowledges what professor of philosophy Gail Weiss says is a recognition of how our bodies are constructed and reconstructed throughout our everyday lives. We have now entered the *sexual ecology* of whole-body sexuality, the reciprocal interpersonal interactions and the interactions between us and our surrounding environment that affect our embodiment of sexuality.

A Phenomenology of Embeddedness

We are essentially embedded within our social and natural environment, meaning we are as much a part of our surroundings as they are a part of us. We live in an ongoing phenomenon of impact and influence. In *Spell of the*

DOI: 10.4324/9780429297236-7

Sensuous, phenomenologist David Abram (1997) describes how "the breathing, sensing body draws its sustenance and its very substance from the soils, plants, and elements that surround it" (pg. 46). To acknowledge that *we are a body* is

> *n*ot to reduce the mystery of my yearnings and fluid thoughts to a set *of mechanisms . . . rather it is to affirm the uncanniness of this physical form. It is not to lock up awareness within the density of a closed and bounded object, for . . . the boundaries of a living body are open and indeterminate; more like membranes than barriers, they define a surface of metamorphosis and exchange. (pg. 46)*

The way that you inhabit your body, your identity, and your sense of self in this moment is a grand co-creation of your complex interface with the natural and human-crafted environment, the people who surround you, and the social institutions that support or exclude you. Our body boundaries are open and permeable and we cannot escape mutual influence. The natural and human-impacted environment influences our pace of life (small town versus city life, for example) as well as physical and mental health. We humans, in turn, impact our environments through everything from agriculture to civic development to oil spills. You may notice that there are certain landscapes that you cannot wait to leave and other landscapes in which you long to be. The social environment even more heavily impacts our behavior and sense of self. Swiss psychotherapist Carl Jung (1952) said that "the meeting of two personalities is like the contact of two chemical substances: if there is any reaction, both are transformed." How I respond to you and how you respond to me impacts us both. Human *intersubjectivity* is a fundamental connecting principle between us and others, forming the building blocks of the social self.

An important mechanism in this co-creation of the self is found between the frontal cortex and limbic system of the brain. Referred to as *mirror neurons*, these specialized brain cells reside within the parietal and premotor cortexes of the brain and they "serve to connect our visual and motor systems with frontal systems responsible for goal-directed behavior" (Cozolino, 2017, pg. 212). These specialized neurons are important because the expressions, the body movements, and the quality of movement effort of others activates our empathy circuits—our brain "lights up" as though we are moving and feeling too. When you witness someone laugh at a joke, cry while in the midst of personal loss, or become angry in response to witnessing the interaction between a surly school bully and a scared classmate, our body responds with sensation and emotion. We learn from how it feels to witness the expression of others and we deduce whether we want to express in the way the others speak or hold their posture based on what resonates with us. This felt experience of witnessing gives us access to *subjective empathy*: experiencing internal sensations and feelings in response to the expression of another. This in turn gives us access to *interpersonal empathy*: the interconnected dance of emotional understanding and mutual influence (Clark, 2010). Upon connecting with another's experience, we can attune with each other, form bonds, and sustain our communities together. Mirror neurons not only facilitate the emotional bonds necessary for our physical and emotional sustenance, they also help us learn about the range of human expression, including what is appropriate to be expressed by us.

Considering that our mirror neurons activate in response to influential people, we can begin to unravel the reasons why we develop such a complex and often sex-negative somatic tapestry of sexuality. As a society, we exchange confusing messages about what sorts of bodies, relationship styles, and sexual expressions are worthy of empathy and attunement. Consider the messages we give and receive about the sexual body when we interact with family, friends, teachers, religious leaders, and media (social media, music videos, pornography, etc.). As people embedded within relational systems, our intersubjective nature determines that the beliefs of the society impact how we organize ourselves internally via our experience-dependent nervous system. As a result, your awareness and experience of your sexual body is deeply impacted by your location within your social and cultural landscape.

Despite cultural change, many of us still live in communities that are largely biased toward heterosexuality, monogamy, and cisgender expression, and there are many people who are immediately excluded and *othered* by these standards. Our culture is at once sex-negative and hypersexualized, thwarting our appreciation of the nuanced erotic self. Any fluctuation in sexual interest or responsiveness is often seen as a problem. Even those who do fit into these categories on the surface silently suffer internally from erotic alienation. We seek to change our bodies, change what we desire, and medically or psychologically treat the parts of ourselves that diverge from those normative standards. In *New Directions in Sex Therapy*, sex therapist and sex researcher Peggy Kleinplatz offers a strong objection to simply treating the symptoms of sexual problems as "technical difficulties, subject to treatment and cure devoid of the psychological, relational and social contexts in which they come to be perceived as problematic" (2012, pg. xxv). Treating symptoms to align with ideal standards often offers only a brief reprieve or creates new problems with which to grapple.

Somatic psychotherapist and author Rae Johnson writes extensively about the pervasive impact of normative sociocultural standards on the somatic self. In Johnson's *Queering/Querying the Body: Sensation and Curiosity in Disrupting Body Norms*, they point out that "almost no one is exempt from ongoing, countless expectations to present our bodily selves in particular ways, and this is especially true for those whose bodies fall outside dominant social norms or whose social position does not afford them the privilege of refusing to conform" (Caldwell & Bennett Leighton, 2018, pg. 98). As the call for awareness and social change mount, we recognize more and more that we are in a collective marginalization and oppression of the erotic body and that this hits marginalized populations the hardest.

We all absorb powerful messages about what sexuality expressions our social position deems appropriate, what types of sexuality are "normal," and what types are not (the "normal" category is more than likely quite narrow and excludes the vast range of what normal actually is). Consider what verbal or nonverbal messages you received and what experiences you had related to sexuality and your body during your formative years. What did you learn about your sexuality based on your gender, your body type, your skin color, your socioeconomic status, your body or cognitive ability, your ethnic group, or your way of dressing? This will begin to give you a sense of your sexual ecology: the social and natural environment in which you were born, in which you grew up, and where you find yourself now.

Cultural Oppression of the Body

Nathaniel Hawthorne's *The Scarlet Letter* offers a vivid example of the impact of a negative sexual environment. The main protagonist, Hester Prynne, is not Puritan herself, yet is shamed and socially stigmatized within a 17th-century Puritan colony for an extramarital relationship and pregnancy. She is ordered to wear a large, red letter "A" on all her clothing, publicly branding her as an *adulteress*. She is scorned and cast aside. Her experience of social alienation causes Hester deep emotional pain and after seven years of social isolation, she loses her warmth and vibrancy—her punishment changes her physical appearance as well as her experience of herself.

This story illustrates how sexual ecology works: we are heavily influenced by our collective experience within agricultural and colonization history. Agricultural practices taught humans how to own and cultivate things, while colonization put the needs and beliefs of an elite few over the rights and needs of the less influential. These combined systems have a sexuality foundation that fractures those who are oppressed by it, as well as those who benefit from it, and this fracture infuses the social layers that surround you at every level—entire systems, communities, families, and your own beliefs.

The "dominant groups get to define which identities are acceptable, and therefore included, and which ones are not, and summarily excluded" (Caldwell & Bennett Leighton, 2018, pg. 34), says somatic psychotherapist Christine Caldwell. When this type of immersive social alienation targets one's sexuality, it creates a fracture through the very source of our generative wellspring, creating an abject or "cast off" part of the erotic self. Can I reach for what I find pleasurable? Can I move, or dress, or love what or who

I love? Can I inhabit my true experience of gender? When we cannot resolve these fundamental questions of embodiment, this fracture is enveloped by protective body armor—bound muscle patterns and hyper-activation of the survival strategy of the nervous system.

The fissure between the socially integrated part of self and the unintegrated, abject part of self can induce a feeling of tension, like rock grinding beneath an earthquake. This enveloping burden presses on the erotic body and pushes it into the shadows of our consciousness and of our society. We then reenact this trauma response on each other through erotic marginalization where we "other," exclude, or punish others for their expression of sexuality. When a family member, teacher, or peer negatively reflects our expression of a pleasurable movement or gender expression, our mirror neurons pick up on their bound or critical response to us and we suppress expression, avoid interaction, or even retaliate.

Each of these moments can become internalized with bound energy in the muscles and pre-effort rhythms (rhythms expressed while learning or defending) in our movements. We store this information in our body landscape, and it becomes integrated with our existing sexual schemas, our beliefs and attitudes about sexuality. The body memories of these difficult moments are later activated by our own arousal or the arousal of another and we experience bound-flow sexual energy, desires marked by guilt, or instability in sexual relationships. Inevitably, we suppress much more than we get to express. In her contribution to *Oppression and the Body*, Lucia Bennett Leighton points out that sociocultural oppression acts like trauma on the body, causing hypervigilance, withdrawal, feeling othered or marginalized, dissociation, and body-based memory that lacks clear cognitive context (Caldwell & Bennett Leighton, 2018). It is difficult to feel fully embodied in our expansive pleasure when we have somatically accumulated more negative or confusing encounters than positive and supportive experiences.

Embodiment, Revisited

When considering the impact of the social environment on our sexuality, we must revisit the concept of *embodiment*. The term itself often shows up in its appropriated form, dressed in the dominant cultural narrative. This is problematic because embodiment is not meant to be a VIP-level experience afforded to the elite few. In speaking about her experience in a black body in the United States, somatic counseling professor and social justice consultant Carla Sherrell expresses that "the demand to simulate white bodies is directly related to the appropriation of the term *embodiment* by whiteness" and that this term "is infused with assumptions of positive outcomes and healing" (Caldwell & Bennett Leighton, 2018, pg. 148). In taking for granted that embodiment is a narrowly defined experience, we minimize the complex reality that people live every day, leaving us with an incomplete picture of a somatic experience. Narrowly defining embodiment also limits our *body autonomy*, the ability to make decisions for our own body, which is respected and upheld by our community.

We all have internalized beliefs from our social environments, and it is beneficial to become aware of harmful or unhelpful ideas that we project onto ourselves or others. For many, especially marginalized people and communities, this is an act of oppression and quickly activates the defenses of the body. Sherrell makes an indispensable point, which can be applied to the healing of sexuality on a somatic level: in our striving for sexual wellness, we must embrace embodiment as a *diverse experience* and we must practice mindful awareness around the judgments we may have about how to inhabit a body, including our own. True embodiment encompasses a vast range of ways to inhabit these diverse and magnificent social bodies. In *Decolonizing Sexualities* (Bakshi, Jivraj, & Posoccco, 2016), Associate Professor of Sociology at Université de Montréal Sirma Bilge emphasizes the importance of making human difference the core of social justice focus and practice. When we protect different forms of embodiment, we have "an invitation to engage difference creatively and generatively, beyond mere tolerance" (pg. 114). Bilge then quotes Audre Lorde's statement that "difference is that raw and powerful connection from which our personal power is forged" (pg. 114).

As we consider the social-ecological reality of ourselves and others, we become better equipped to see the ways we were taught to contain ourselves in order to keep secret our desires, our curiosities, and our vivid creativity. As we increase awareness, we access the ability to unwind negative beliefs, appreciate our intelligent protective mechanisms, and refine how to embody erotic vitality, just as you are, in the social spaces where it feels safe enough to do so. Embodiment of sexuality does not just represent primarily able-bodied and joyful expressiveness. The cultivation of embodiment does not require that we relinquish our protective body armor, our unique quirks and ways of expressing, or our kinky interests. Embodiment is quite simply (though not easily) the act of intentionally making visible what is internal.

Social-Sexual Ecology

When we look at a social-sexual environment, we look at the features of an individual such as race, ethnicity, gender presentation and gender assignment, body ability, age, socioeconomic class, and beliefs. Then we look at the interplay between their individual features and the features of their family, their community, and their society to better understand their experience and expression.

Your social ecology looks like this (Figure 6.1):

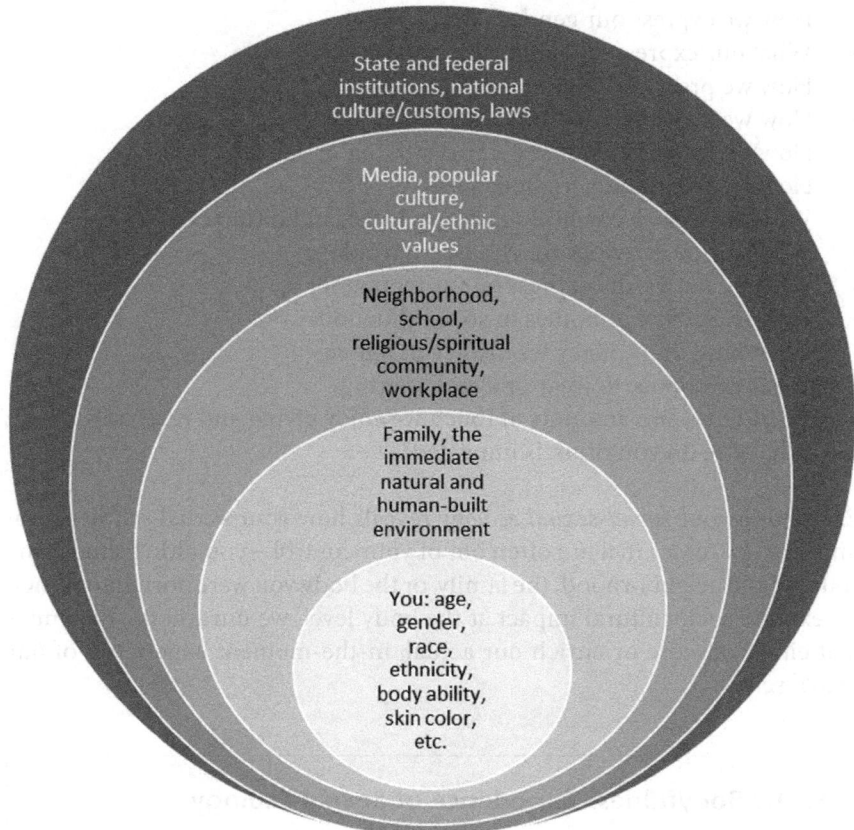

Figure 6.1 Social Ecology Impacting Embodiment of Sexuality

Everything, from language to body posture and movement, from the identity that we express and the identity that we keep secret, is a convergence of genetics and experiences at these levels of social structure. Your sexuality does not escape this confluence. When we apply this perspective to our sexual development, we see how the verbal and nonverbal messages from family, community, and society have made their impact on sexuality experience and expression. These messages and direct experiences affect how we feel in our bodies, how we sense and express our arousal, what beliefs we have formed around sex, and what assumptions we make about the sexuality of others. Our social and cultural upbringing impacts:

- What we learned about sex, reproductive, and arousal anatomy
- How we have sex
- How we are assigned a gender

- How we express our gender
- What our expressed relationship style is
- How we practice active consent (or not)
- How we feel about and treat our body
- How we feel about our sexual orientation
- How we communicate about sex
- What we feel we can give or receive in sex and intimacy
- What sexual activities we choose or avoid
- Who we outwardly express our attraction for
- How we move our bodies in social situations
- What kind of intimacy we display in public
- What we choose to wear or avoid wearing
- What types and amounts of touch we enjoy giving and receiving
- What else do you think is impacted?

Examining your *social-sexual ecology* reveals how your sexual self has been impacted by forces that are often out of your control—you didn't choose the country, the neighborhood, the family, or the body you were born into. When we explore sociocultural impact at the body level, we unravel the dynamics that either obscure or enrich our actual, in-the-moment experience of our sexual selves.

Erotic Bodyfulness Experience of Sexual Ecology

Review the social-sexual ecology image (Figure 6.1) and begin at the center circle. Notice your internal felt sense and movement signature in this moment as a baseline. Then notice how your baseline felt sense and movement/posture experience changes when you consider the messages about sex and sexuality received from your family. Move on to the next layer and notice your internal and expressive experience when considering the messages from your surrounding communities. Now notice your felt sense and movement expression when considering the messages you received from the larger cultural influences like the media and dominant cultural or national values. Notice which social layers and specific messages cause your body to constrict, twist away uncomfortably, restrict your breath, shrink your posture. Also notice which social layers and messages invite you to open, expand, soften, and allow for excitement and dynamic movement. As you explore your social-sexual ecology through this somatic lens, notice how your breath, body sensations, movements and gestures, posture, and eye contact shifts. Noticing the posture and gesture of the body gives us a direct language of the impact our environment has on our implicit ways of being in the world.

When Opal entered my office to work on her inability to orgasm with a partner, she was confounded. "Why can I orgasm on my own—no problem—but when I have sex with a partner I just can't get there no matter how much stimulation or time we take?" We explored Opal's experience and found that her awareness became heavily external when she was engaging sexually with someone else. She focused everywhere but on her own sensations—she noticed her partner looking at her body, she noticed how her body position emphasized certain features, she made sure she was making pleasurable sounds, etc.

As she recounted her last sexual encounter, Opal reported very little sensation in her body and her breath being caught in her upper chest and throat. I asked Opal what the constricted breath in her upper chest was trying to do for her—what job does it think it has to do? "It's helping me make sure that I look good, because if I don't look good or sound like I'm enjoying myself, I might be criticized." Whoa. "Does this feel familiar?" I ask. We began to explore her sexual ecology and the messages she received about sexuality and her body from her family. Opal described her experience in her family. "My dad often commented on how other women looked, including my mom and me and sisters, and would criticize us for our bodies or the way we moved. I really wanted my dad's approval, and I thought that if I got it right, he'd stop criticizing me. As a Japanese-American family in a very white town, I know that my dad was really aware of our appearance and didn't want me and my sisters to get bullied too much. We got bullied anyway. Between the criticism I got at school and the criticism I got from my dad, it was better to not feel too much."

Opal's experience with her dad and with her school fellows made a deep impact on how she felt about her body, how she carried herself, and how she connected with her ability to feel pleasure with a sexual partner. Combine this with the messages she received from a media culture which is hyper-focused on how a woman looks, and we have a recipe for orgasm-suppression. Her experience of her family and community dynamic and the broader media culture had written itself directly on her somatic nervous system and arousal anatomy by hyper-externalizing her awareness. By numbing her authentic sensations, movements, and sounds, she felt safer, even though it created a numbing buffer between herself and her embodied expression of pleasure.

Emerging From the Cultural Trenches

What presents us with the greatest challenges in life also has the potential to gift us with our greatest superpower. As you begin to somatically explore the social and cultural influences that have *othered* you in some way, look for your strength and appreciate the ways that your somatic self has protected you by diverting your creative energies. Perhaps you felt you couldn't express your sexuality in a particular way, but you could dance like a badass, so you channeled your erotic vitality into your art. While exploring your sexual ecology, you can harvest the social messages and experiences that have supported the emerging embodiment of your creativity and magnificence.

Amplifying our attention on the somatic experience of support from sexuality allies interrupts the habituated defensive movements while bolstering what allows us to appreciate and embody sexuality. These are our internal resources acquired from outside supports. Maybe you came across an interview with Dr. Ruth in which this renowned sex-positive advocate extolled the normalcy and beauty of sex. Maybe you had an aunt who was unabashedly direct as she passed on wisdom about menstruation and personal hygiene. Or maybe you had a core group of friends that excitedly helped you change your wardrobe when you transitioned your gender identity. When I work with my clients, I invite them to explore these positive verbal and nonverbal sexual messages that they have received and, using erotic bodyfulness, notice the in-the-moment somatic impact of these external sources. How did it feel somatically as your aunt calmly talked to you about menstruation or when your friends hugged you when you found the perfect outfit? This allows my clients to pan for gold—to sift through the inaccurate and unhelpful assessments of their desires to find the gems, the positive moments, just waiting to be polished and set out in the sun to reflect our light.

As we are infused with the messages of our sexuality allies, the way is cleared to explore the true nature of what sparks arousal and interest. Once the gems are discovered, invite fantasy or real-world exploration to allow the organicity (growth orientation) of the desire to catch up to your current self. Over time and repetition, the discovery of vitality allows the opportunity to heal the vestiges of familial and social wounds that we carry.

Erotic Bodyfulness Experience of Sexual Allyship

Remember a moment when you felt supported in your sexuality by a friend, a lover, or even a character in a movie. Notice your felt sense and movement expression that begins to happen within and around your somatic landscape. Allow yourself to exaggerate the movements that you feel coming from within and notice the qualities of the movements that are outwardly expressed. Invite your breath to support and extend the movements directly from the source of the sensation in your body. A deeper in-breath and longer out-breath increases sensation and use of kinesphere (the space that your body can take up). As you explore and repeat the movements, notice how your internal felt sense experience becomes amplified. Do another body scan to check in with what may feel different within your somatic landscape. What are the affirming messages that your body is communicating to you now?

Remember, it's okay if you still sense your body armor or a hesitance to express a broader range of movement. This is a practice of appreciating your complexity while intentionally acting from a place of self-affirmation to the best of your ability given the context that you are in. When you feel safe enough (just enough safety to take a risk in sharing a tender part of yourself), responding from a self-affirming place will be just a bit easier.

Make a few notes of the sensations and movement qualities and take a few moments to validate your emotional response to embodying the movements of feeling supported. You may be surprised to find a mixture of emotions (for example, comfort and sadness). Allow the space for your emotion as you return to your prior movements. As you continue to move, you may notice a change in your emotional quality. Emotions that are literally moved (the Latin root of emotion is "to move") have an opportunity to unwind the bound muscle tension that keeps body armor in place.

Now what do you notice?

Mirrors to Our Beauty: The Role of Community in Embodied Sexuality

One of the most important topics in sexuality work is the vital role that community plays in sexual healing. Your supportive community can consist of friends, family, lovers or committed partners, a therapist or coach, a kink community, a spiritual community, a cuddle group, a dance group, a therapeutic support group, or an online community, just to name a few. Just as we would travel to Portugal to immerse ourselves in Portuguese language and culture, your community can provide a space for you to practice speaking the mother-tongue language of the body in real-time relationship. As we unwind relational and social wounds, dispelling incorrect beliefs and assumptions, the community that you choose can have a profound impact on the longevity of your personal work. Your community provides connection, reciprocity, bonding, shared experience, shared values, and exploratory play. They cheer you on, tell you that you are beautiful or brave, resonate with stories, practice attunement, explore new sexual play, and so much more. Affirming messages about your sexuality, they help you begin to dethrone the old, invalidating messages.

While wounding happens in relationship, healing also happens in relationship. This is the principle of rupture and repair, of witnessing and being witnessed, that gives the opportunity for a reparative experience. Witnessing others as they witness us in a supportive, co-creative spirit offers us an opportunity to see ourselves through the eyes of an encouraging person and to learn of a potential that we have not yet dreamed. Remember those mirror neurons? New ways of moving, accessing pleasure, setting boundaries, and more can be learned in relationship. In my workshops, I facilitate many witnessing experiences because it gives my participants an opportunity to activate the mirror neurons of the brain, stimulating both brain rewiring and the expansion of our movement repertoire. Our current community offers an opportunity to repair the attachment wounds that inevitably form from our younger years, expanding our movement potential and generating more positive self-talk.

Fundamentally, community helps us to not feel alone, to feel appreciated and wanted just as we are, in both our learning and our mastery. When conflict or disagreement arises, community allows us the opportunity to practice repair as we self-regulate and maintain connection with our somatic selves. How we embody our inner selves is heavily dependent on context. Based on our social-sexual location, it may or may not be appropriate, or even safe, to fully express ourselves. A good community can help us feel safe enough to practice being vulnerable so that we may heal the fractures from a sex-negative social environment to find ground in our vulnerability and transparency.

7

EROTIC ON THE OUTSIDE

Expressing a Whole-Body Sexuality

I crouch on the floor of the dance studio, my limbs tightly curled around my core like a flower bud as I am guided by my Butoh instructor, Maureen Momo Freehill, to embody a flower at three different stages. Butoh, a dance form rooted in a dramatic expression of the human condition, often explores life and death cycles in vivid and exaggerated movements of the face and body. In the first stage of our exploration, we are a flower just beginning to open its petals toward the sun. I push my feet into the floor while tentatively reaching my spine toward the sun, my arms softly wrapped around my body-stem as my heart just peeks open to detect the warmth with new delight. I feel my sequencing has just begun, not ready to fully extend. The sun sets and I descend back into a tightly wrapped flower bud.

In the second stage, Freehill tells us we are flowers in our full daylight glory. With new confidence, I again push into the floor with my feet, pelvis rising as my spine and arms unfurl, opening my petals wide as I soak up the delicious sunlight. My pelvic floor softens above the warm ground as my chest and face rise up directly from my core to sway and hover in the air, luscious and languid. The endpoints of my body—hands and feet, tailbone, and crown of my head—extend to the fullest point of my reach. I can feel the very fascia of my body, that full-body sheet of connective tissue, stretching taught at my growing edge. Then sun sets and I descend back into the sleeping flower, arms wrapped like petals around my ribs.

Freehill then announces the third and final stage where we know this will be our last time in the sun before our petals fall to the ground to make room for new life. With confidence and bittersweet sadness in my chest, a layer of aching grief just below my skin, I push my feet into the floor for the last time, much more slowly than before, savoring every inch as I rise and unfurl

DOI: 10.4324/9780429297236-8

my softened petals. I hover, almost grasping and gulping the sun and then I descend, laying on the floor in the full, active release of yield.

Freehill's "Three Days of the Flower" (Baird and Candelario, 2018) is used as an exploration of the full spectrum of the embodied human condition. I have experienced this dynamic fullness of expression in other areas of my life, such as the coordination of flow in my arms with hip articulations while belly dancing and when interacting in play with my intimate partner.

This is what dance/movement therapists would call an exploration of pre-effort to full-effort movement sequence—a skillfully coordinated series of movements toward actualizing a clear purpose: to better know my own growth and longing through the life cycle of a flower.

In *Mozart in the Jungle*, we see this fullness of body connection when maestro Rodrigo DeSousa identifies musicians who "play with the blood." In the series, we learn that this phrase emerged from his experience of playing the violin so precisely and passionately, so fully caught up in the moment, that his fingers bled from their dance with the strings. While some musicians simply play the notes on the page, the maestro is entranced by those who *become the music* and express so passionately that they literally bleed on the strings of their instrument. In the dance/movement therapy practice of Authentic Movement, we call this *moving and being moved* at the same time. We are not simply "going through the motions"; we are moving in amorous synchrony with ourselves. It is that effortless edge of expression where we trust our body enough to let it move us, unhindered by the judging mind.

Based on our embedded experience within family and surrounding culture, our individual expression looks and feels essentially different from each other, yet there are similar fundamental elements that we can identify and refine. Namely, we can explore body (the internal landscape experience), effort (the qualities of movement), shape (how the body changes shape in space), and space (where the body moves and what inspires it to do so) to support full body expression.

It is of vital importance that, as we go forward, sensing and assessing your range of movement repertoire is done *without comparing yourself to anyone else*. This is not a competition of how overtly expressive or vocal we can be in our erotic selves. Instead, this is about unearthing the fullness of *your* potential. This chapter is a guide to help you reach deeply within yourself, connect with your sensation, and express your sexuality directly from the core of your sensory aliveness. Expressive erotic fullness can exist in the smallest and most imperceptible of movements (micro-movements). Regardless of age, body type, or ability, the moving erotic body is the phenomenological playground for experience and relationship.

Erotic expression is also not about expressing just for the benefit of others, to live up to some imagined ideal, or to change who we are. By sequencing movement through the interconnectivity of the body, sensation is heightened, pulling on us to connect with our actual, in-the-moment potential. *We become more of who we already are.* Let's explore the elements of full-effort movement in the realm of the erotic.

Unearthing this potential, no matter your body ability, is possible because sexuality *is* the moving body. In *Sensuality and the Dance* (1983), choreographer Sheldon Ossosky said "the body [is] basically sensual . . . sexuality results from the way this sensual body is used" (p. 5). In class, Ossosky would facilitate his dancers in movement explorations via sensual imagery, similar to my Butoh instructor, inviting his dancers to embody more of their embodied vitality and erotic fullness. This technique produced more expressive and palpable dancers, moving from the inside out instead of simply replicating choreography.

Ossossky's process relates directly to the practice of erotic bodyfulness, which helps us become aware of the matrix of our unique internal erotic map as well as how we project the embedded erotic body-mind dynamic through small and large gestures and in relationship with breath, voice tone and pitch, and posture. Movement is symbolic and it is also our lived stories in motion, sometimes practical, sometimes profound. Movement can indicate and express everything from emotion to gender identity. Jane Desmond (2001), professor of anthropology and gender studies, and former modern dancer, indicates in *Dancing Desires* that "how one moves, and how one moves in relation to others, constitutes a public enactment of sexuality and gender" (pg. 6). Desmond encourages an exploration of the kinesthetics of sexuality through dance and movement in order to truly understand how sexuality is inhabited, embodied, and experienced.

Our movement qualities also aid us in amplifying the sensations of the body, both to heighten and to mute, to extend and expand pleasure or to minimize pleasure. A vital component of exploring sexuality on a somatic level is to identify the movement qualities in our erotic lives, to feel the impact of our movement qualities internally, and to learn what our movements are communicating to others. From here, we can deepen and refine erotic expression with increased whole-body awareness and embodied erotic intelligence. Let's explore how your movement impacts both your sense of yourself and your expression to others.

Body Talk

Consider the movement qualities that you express in sex—in solo sex, in partner sex, as well as within the whole range of intimacy (cuddling, holding hands, facial expression during emotion, etc.). How much breath fills your body? How much of your body do you move during sex and intimacy? By move, I don't necessarily mean gesturing and moving every part of your body. Do you express the more indulging types of movement: a deep breath, an elongated torso, a softly opened mouth? This is the type of movement that knows the space is safe enough and fascinating enough to expand into and explore with the skin, hips, hands. Do you express the more assertive and direct types of movement? The *fighting* rhythms in dance/movement therapy are about penetrating the space and making an impact, which releases endorphins and increases excitement. Or do you find that your movement is minimal or localized? This type of bipolar (both sides of the body) or unipolar (one side of the body) *narrowing* movement is marked by the body following a patterned sequence—like an established path, movement has little feeling and nuance and is rigid and predictable. The narrower movements can become a choreographed dance—boring but efficient and either gets the job done or simply gets it over quickly. Even when we want to express more fully, we can become stuck in the rigid pattern. Do you find your movement to be more chaotic, with overflowing boundaries, and lacking present moment awareness and self-directed containment? This movement style denotes too much free-flow energy and could be a sign of dissociation, lack of impulse control, or blissfully depersonalized transcendence.

You can experience all of these movement profiles depending on the context or intrapersonal factors like mood, interest, or sense of safety. Each of us has a choreography of movement signatures that speak their truth and present us with an opportunity for call and response—a call to the pressure points of the body for us to press into and address underlying needs and imbalances. The movement signatures that we inhabit are also carried forward from our family and lineage, continuing a story and a tradition that we inherit. This movement signature is uploaded into the core of the self and becomes a lens through which we see and interpret the world as well as a lens through which others experience us. By exploring our own movement story and giving our own language to it, we have the option to change the tradition of what we communicate and pass on to others that does not support embodiment. Like Kevin Bacon in *Footloose* (1984), we can bring dancing back to a sensually rigid town. We can expand our movement repertoire (the expressive options available to us) as well as impact how we feel in our bodies.

We are too often embedded within a limiting and shaming paradigm of sexuality. As a result, so many of us are stuck in the uncertainty of *pre-effort* movements, which are movement qualities expressed while learning or defending. Pre-effort movements are on their way to mastery, but by definition remain unskilled, half-hearted, overdone, and/or disorganized and distracted. They arise from a place of learning something new or defending against something unwelcome. Like a young child learning to ride a bike without training wheels for the first time, we are wide-eyed and wobbly. When pre-effort movement is dominant, sensation is quarantined to minimal areas of the body or diffuse and disorganized and therefore sex is minimally satisfying, if satisfying at all. During solo sex, we can become hyper-focused on genitals and on orgasm, thereby narrowing movement and excluding the whole of the somatic landscape. Sometimes efficiency is exactly what we need, but too much efficiency minimizes our erotic potential and pleasure possibility. During partnered sex, one can sense the repeated sequence, the hesitancy, the closed expression and therefore withhold parts of themselves in return or blow past boundaries they may or may not realize are being crossed. Sex is such a secret and taboo area of life that we often walk around in a state of sexual pre-effort—still trying to figure out how to ride the bike while defending against running our bike into others or being run over ourselves. We are not sure how to be sexual or how to express ourselves sexually. We avoid certain sexual behavior, sexual situations, or sexual relationships altogether.

Full-effort embodiment takes time to develop, but we often don't allow ourselves the time to do this and then judge ourselves for what we perceive to be flaws in our sexuality or sexual responsiveness. Somehow, whether through peers or media, we learn that we should be sex experts as adults even though we have been restricted from accurate and inclusive information as young ones. "It should just be natural," I hear so many clients say. The places to gather good sexual information are rare and woefully inadequate—we get silence, sterile medical information, or curated sexual videos of actors *performing* sexual behavior. Meanwhile, the abundance of sex-negative experiences pushes us to fear most things about sex. This is not a good setup for learning the embodied, full-effort sex that lifts us up and deepens our connection with a partner. As sex and relationship therapist Esther Perel says, "It has to be sex worth wanting," and pre-effort sex is what brings clients to my couch. Only if sex is practiced, explored, and supported will it be sex worth having.

For many, limiting sexual expression to a pre-effort activity is a survival skill that had been supportive, even necessary at one point, yet currently detracts from accessing fully satisfying erotic lives. Even if we feel the fullness of sensation, shaming or unsafe experiences may muddy the waters and cause us to retract from that sensation.

Both pre-effort and full-effort expressions are not necessarily found exclusively without the other—they work in concert. We are always learning and integrating new experiences, even when we express mastery. Just as our muscles flex and release in a symphony of bound- and free-flow tension to create body movements, full effort and pre-effort work together to navigate the challenges of our changing environment. An important component of developing more full-bodied sexuality is the practice of listening to the language of the pre-effort expression and letting it be awkward and uncoordinated in order to learn what is needed to expand into increased confidence and mastery.

Dissonant Desire

While exploring their sexual relationship, a client recently lamented, "I feel an intensity of ten on the inside, but it looks like a four to my partner. They can't tell that I'm into it at all." This client had developed an erotic expressiveness marked by a bound emotional and somatic presence. They did not feel safe enough to express the fullness of their internal experience, so they had developed body armor to contain and mute their intensity. The muting of expression can also happen over the course of a relationship as partners become more complacent with each other.

As I explore with my clients the movement qualities that emerge as they speak about their sex lives or as a couple co-creates a somatic sculpture in the middle of my office floor, something peculiar happens repeatedly: their bodies send what looks like glaringly conflicting messages. Of course, this is so. Like running pasta through a clogged spiralizer, our sexual energy gets distorted or changes shape based on the relational and cultural filters that have formed in our muscles, soft tissues, and body structure.

About one month into our work, Catherine and Tara co-created a somatic sculpture in my office to explore how they felt about their sexual relationship after some initial repair work. Tara, a Latinx professional athlete, had been habitually putting Catherine first, focusing on pleasuring Catherine, never asking for what she wanted. For Catherine, this meant a laser focus on her sexual responsiveness, which induced a hollowing of her chest and increased bound flow in her pelvis, as though her arousal anatomy was shrinking from being seen. Catherine, a white marketing specialist from the Midwest, valued her ability to please her partners. For her, this lack of arousal with Tara was maddening. She loved and felt attraction for Tara, and Catherine wanted so much for her desire to respond in kind. We decided to explore what, on the surface, looked like "mixed messages." As they stood facing each other, I invited Tara to soften her pelvis with a slight backward tilt as her knees bent and her arms opened toward Catherine. Meanwhile, Catherine stepped closer to Tara, feeling the pull to be closer, while simultaneously leaning her shoulders back with chin pulled in, jaw set, and eyes squinted as she searched Tara's face and body. I noticed that, as Catherine's eyes contracted, Tara's chest retracted just slightly. "I just don't know if she actually wants me. It was you who told her to soften," Catherine said immediately, subtly contracting in her midline and almost imperceptibly rounding her shoulders. "Does this feel familiar to you?" I asked them. "Yes," they both replied in unison. Catherine turned her gaze to me. "I feel flustered and exhausted by this," she said.

I invited Catherine to close her eyes and rest as I encouraged Tara to enhance the slight contraction that she felt, to follow this movement impulse and learn where it wanted to take her. "I feel judged," she said, placing her hands over her chest, "and I want to hide. Even though I feel warmth in my pelvis, I'm starting to feel that shield over my chest." I invited Tara to close her eyes as I turned back to Catherine, guiding her to focus on her out-breath, shift her weight into her heels, and breathe into her back body (sacrum, spine, back of the skull). I saw the muscles around her eyes soften and I guided her to again see her partner, finding something to breathe in about Tara that she absolutely loved. When Tara opened her eyes again to connect with Catherine, both partners smiled and simultaneously stepped a little closer to each other. From here, I encouraged Tara to invite sensual contact from Catherine as Catherine worked to again breathe into her back body as she offered contact and received Tara's pleasurable response to a hand on her hip. At this point the attunement of their sensual connection with each other was palpable.

When we can identify a quality of expression or touch that is communicating a hesitant or limiting belief about our sexual self, a pathway to transform how our bodies relate erotically to others is uncovered. When we can identify a narrowing in one part of the body with a widening in another, we can invite congruence into a body that is communicating the complex pleasure response of wanting two different things at once. Sometimes this is about wanting to connect intimately but having other responsibilities to attend to. Other times, this arousal non-concordance expresses that the mind wants sex but the body cannot become aroused or the body wants sex while the mind is unsure. This can also be a simultaneous desire for intimacy and connection while being unsure if one "deserves" pleasure, or if a partner truly desires them, or if the person(s) they are with is someone that they want to be sexual with. The examples in the complexity of the "yes" and the "no" are as endless as there are human beings. And in none of these cases is the answer to override the "yes" or the "no"; this is an invitation to slow down and attend to what the expressive erotic body is communicating.

Arousal non-concordance is common, normal, and a call to lean into yourself and breathe some compassion around your challenge. This is about linking up your internal awareness of your sexual self with your interpersonal expressiveness—how the inside responds to and expresses within the intimate relational field—and how expression itself impacts how we experience our body and our sexuality. We come full circle with Irmgard Bartenieff's "lively interplay between internal connectivity and external expressivity" (Hackney, 2003, pg. 34) and we get to see and feel our wholeness represented in the kinesphere of space that surrounds each and every body.

Moving Into Erotic Expressiveness

Erotic expression is about connecting with our body in a way that volumizes our pleasurable lived experience. Full-effort erotic expressiveness is a layered process. When we refine one aspect of sexuality, this unlocks another area we can learn about and venture into. Unlocking our growing edges of expressiveness also encourages us to access deeper levels of what we've already mastered, especially when we begin to embody our sexual selves in other contexts (for example, sex with new lovers, gender expression at work, or going dancing with a new friend group). Life offers endless opportunities to apply and share our erotic intelligence. Knowing the fundamentals of embodied expression is a useful tool along the way.

Erotic expression is also about volumizing our emotional body. Restrictive body postures cause us to feel personally restricted, angry, depressed, or even hopeless (Briñol, Petty, & Wagner, 2009). When speaking about sex, many of my clients adopt rounded postures and tighter voices, literally dropping into less expressive and pre-effort states. Open and expansive body postures, however, cause us to feel confident and hopeful. At a 2019 training in Denver, Colorado, sex educator Emily Nagoski talked about "exhausting" emotions through the body, allowing them to move all the way through their desired expression, thereby clearing our internal pipes for pleasurable feelings and warm connection with others. Movement becomes the broom that sweeps out the cobwebbed corners of our body as the bristles tingle our skin to life.

The Elements of Full-Effort Erotic Expressiveness

Full-effort movements are fueled by the breath and start from the core of the body or the core of sensation with dynamic alignment, the urge to move into space, and perhaps even reach out to touch another. Just as a dancer refines and conditions their body to not simply make shapes but to *embody* movement and the transitions between movement with full-body connectivity, this section will guide you through the process of exploring how *your* body can express your full effort sexuality within your kinesphere. Kinesphere is a concept created by Rudolf Laban, dance artist and movement theorist, to describe "the sphere around the body whose periphery can be reached by easily extended limbs without stepping away from that place which is the point of support when standing on one foot" (Laban, 1974, pg. 10). To Laban, external movement patterns and use of space had parallels to different ways of thinking. Let's explore each element through the fundamental principles of total-body connectivity as articulated by movement analyst Peggy Hackney and her mentor Irmgard Bartenieff.

Breath Support

Breath is the foundational life-giving force of our body—it is vitality itself. International Laban/Bartenieff movement analyst Peggy Hackney says that breath "is the key to life, movement, and rhythm" (2003, pg. 51). Breath initiates and underlies movement—it increases sensation and awareness by opening muscles and submerging interoceptive nerve cells with blood and oxygen, increases power and strength behind movements, releases tension with a long and slow or a fast and vigorous out-breath, and supports the expression and sequencing of emotion.

By allowing your breath to inform how you inhabit your body, it can reveal what muscles and body postures need in the way of adjustment to make room for the fullness that the body desires. By listening closely, your breath will tell you to soften and open your shoulders, to slightly bend your knees and gently tilt your pelvis, to expand and soften the muscles around your eyes, or to shake off physical or emotional tension to make room for more ease of breath.

Without breath support, movement can feel hollow and tangential, a restricted and unsupported reach from the periphery of the body. To a partner, movement can feel uncertain, hesitant, even jarring. As we notice movement impulses arising during erotic bodyfulness practice, your breath becomes the energetic catalyst to support a movement impulse to unfold with grounded intention and satisfying fullness.

Erotic Bodyfulness Experiment With Breath Support

Take a moment now to drop your awareness into your body. Before you take a full breath, notice the sensation qualities in your somatic landscape (temperature, texture, movement). Now, invite three full-body breaths. Let the in-breath expand the whole of your body—your rib cage, diaphragm, belly, pelvis, and limbs—allowing every cell to breathe at once. This is called cellular breathing. Meanwhile, your out-breath softens your body as a whole. Allow your body to shift and adjust to make room for the breath to fill you up. Shift your pelvis, lengthen your spine, roll your shoulders back, or roll your neck. Do whatever your body is asking for to increase the internal space that your breath touches.

After the three full breaths, let the awareness of your body tell you about its landscape now. What is the same and what is different? If you notice a movement impulse—to release your shoulders, stretch your limbs, reach for a drink—surround the sensation of movement impulse with breath and then follow the movement directive.

Next, engage in something pleasurable like dancing, lying in the sun, or a sexual activity. As you engage in this activity, notice the experience of your somatic landscape followed by inviting in those three full-body cellular breaths. Do a body scan and find a place in your body that is experiencing pleasure. Surround this pleasurable sensation with breath and notice a movement impulse that has its origins here at the core of the sensation. Let your in-breath support you as you slowly follow this internal movement directive. Do one more body scan to notice the impact of this breath support. What is the same; what is different?

If you do not notice pleasure but instead notice discomfort or pain, surround this area with breath and allow it with a strong out-breath. We are not trying to change the experience of the body but are simply giving it more space. After your full breath, notice again if anything is different.

Sequencing From Impulse and Core Connectivity

The second element of erotic expressivity is the process of initiating movement from the core of the body (the pelvic and lower belly area) and sequencing it to its full expression and extension, all the way through our endpoints (hands, feet, head, and tail or pelvic floor) for total-body connectivity. The sequenced movement can be large and obvious or subtle and almost imperceptible. The movement impulses that initiate a sequence have a trajectory that is somatically intelligent and speaks to us of our underlying needs, desires, and energetic personality. By encouraging movement to play out with the help of breath support, we neurophysiologically link up our body's connectivity through all the pathways between our core and distal endpoints. These pathways have roots in our earliest development and form the underlying architecture of expression. The pathway of *naval radiation* is when movement is initiated and extends from the core of our body as seen in the belly breath and jellyfish-like contraction and expansion of the body as a whole; the pathway of *core/distal* connectivity is movement that travels from the core into the hands, feet, tailbone, and head of the body in precise articulation; the pathway of *head-tail* connectivity allows for the coordinated movement from the top of the spine to bottom of spine like when we elongate the torso to sit up straight; the pathway of *upper-lower* connection allows the body to yield in to active rest, and push, then reach and pull with balance and strength; the pathway of *body-half* connection allows side-to-side movement sequencing like crawling or walking; and finally, the pathway of *cross-lateral* connection creates the diagonal pathways through the body, allowing for awareness and movement that travels across the body as in counterbalancing with the left lower body to reach up and diagonally to the right to grab something off a high shelf (Hackney, 2003).

We are often attracted to those who move with total-body connectivity as it presents an embodiment of confidence and clarity of purpose. When we connect our movement impulses from the core of the body to our breath, the outcome is a movement sequence characterized by a fullness and clarity that is both satisfying and attractive. Regardless of physical ability, those who are confident move from the inside out and allow their physical and verbal movements to progress to fill up the space around them.

Because breath and movement increase sensation, sequencing movement from our core to our endpoints amplifies our sensory range and potential. We feel pleasure more deeply and in more areas of our body. From the bowl of our pelvis and its extensive network of arousal anatomy, we carve through the space, molding and contouring our body in a sensual, voluminous dance with our own body or with the body of a lover or lovers.

Movement can also emerge from a sensation and then move out through the endpoints. With breath support we can locate pleasurable sensations, heighten them, release tension, and acknowledge a movement impulse to follow directly from the origin point of the sensation itself. Embodied erotic expressiveness is a validation and reification of one's own pleasure and desire—we value our pleasure and listen with curiosity and interest to what it can teach us. By inviting pleasure-initiated movement, we allow our desires and sexual energy to complete a developmental and even evolutionary cycle. We invite the mastery that unlocks further aspects of the sexual self.

Additionally, movement can begin from the core of the body or sensation out through the vocal cords in the form of sound, audible breath, or words. When we sound and speak from our core, our communication is sourced directly from our desire or from our boundaries. For example, based on where within the body we are speaking from, our paraverbals (tone, pitch, volume) can communicate important information about what we tell our lovers. Try tightening the muscles of your core and rib cage and saying, "I want you." What is the underlying message that you just communicated? Then, soften your body and breathe into your belly and pelvis, and say, "I want you." Now what do you feel you communicated? Notice how the tone of your muscles impacted the origin and quality of your tone.

Erotic Bodyfulness Experiment With Sequencing From Core Connectivity

Visualize something that you find pleasurable. Engage your breath and allow any body adjustments you need so you can breathe fully. Breathe around a pleasurable sensation—a warmth in your belly, thickness in your erectile tissue (everyone has erectile tissue), a fluttering just under your diaphragm—and soften your pelvic floor muscles to invite your breath to fill your pelvic bowl. Sink into this moment. As you focus on this pleasurable sensation, listen for the movement impulse but do not yet follow this impulse. Do you notice a trajectory, a rhythm that calls you to move? Now, slowly and with full breath, allow your body to unfold toward the movement impulse. One. Delicious. Increment. At a time. Follow the pace and network of your connective tissues, the fascia and tissues between your larger muscles, until the movement extends all the way through your hands, or feet, or head, or pelvic floor.

Sequencing through the endpoints may not be the end of the movement. Listen for a rhythm or repetition that wants to happen and continue to slowly follow as a rhythm builds. Remember to breathe. You may catch your breath at certain locations in your body. Make note of these locations where breath becomes stuck—these are the landmarks of stuck energy. Don't rush through the stuck places—these are places

> *where body armor is protecting something, so listen to the quality of stuckness and what it is telling you. Repeat your movement sequence as slowly as you can until you can more smoothly transition through these obstructions.*
>
> *Slow your movement and bring your awareness back to the point of origin of the impulse. Has the sensation changed? Has the desired movement changed? Follow the next movement impulse by sinking into your core and sequencing through the endpoints once again.*

Dynamic Alignment

Like a spiral staircase, the spine coils upward as you look over your shoulder at your lover—a twisting body rhythm signals a flirtatious invitation. Spinning kicks transition into fluid hip undulations by the Fly Girls in the '90s comedy show *In Living Color*. We can shift between slow and sensual to passionate or to impact play in sex. We can indulge and open to the "yes" of pleasure exchange, then shift into a retracted "no" when pleasure is displaced by discomfort. Due to the complexity of our skeletal, muscular, and tissue structures, we have the refined ability to quickly shift directions, balance ourselves on uncertain terrain, and respond to the ever-morphing demands presented by the environments in which our somatic selves are embedded. This is the robust quality of dynamic alignment—the body intelligence of balance through moment-to-moment adaptability.

Dynamic alignment is beautifully demonstrated in the subtle contact improvisation practice of the *small dance*. Originated by American dancer and choreographer Steve Paxton, contact improvisation is primarily a dance done in relationship to others that focuses on the bodily sharing of weight, touch, and movement awareness. The *small dance* is a solo body awareness exploration in preparation for interpersonal movement. This fundamental practice brings awareness to how the body dynamically responds to the impact of gravity. Even in stillness, we are never static. When we stand, extending up over our stacked feet and hips, we can perceive the multitude of tiny bony and muscular adjustments made from the top of the spine all the way down to the sacrum, knees, and feet, which keep us standing in the vertical position. These many almost imperceptible movements in concert are the building blocks that merge into the experience of balance. If someone were to gently push us while standing, dynamic alignment is what allows us to absorb the push and return to vertical integrity.

In sexuality, it is dynamic alignment that makes the sequencing of movement possible as we express or sequester our arousal energy. It allows us to navigate between our desires and the desires of a lover.

Erotic Bodyfulness Experiment With Dynamic Alignment

You can either stand or sit for this experiment, though most of the guidance will assume standing. If you are sitting, allow your feet to rest flat in front of you to the best of your ability as you connect as much of your pelvic floor (bottom of your pelvis) as possible to the seat beneath you. Do not rest your spine into the back of your seat, if possible. If standing, stand with your feet just hip-distance apart, knees slightly bent, and your arms resting long at your sides. Stand as still as possible and invite three full-body breaths. Open the awareness coming from your feet. Notice how your feet respond to being the base of your entire body as your mass presses up against the force of gravity. Do you notice the slight shift between your heels, the large joint that connects your big toe to your foot, and the small joint that connects your smallest toe to your foot? These three points create a triangle. Do you notice how your weight shifts between these three points? Invite the awareness of the muscles in your legs. Notice how your body sways gently as you stand, engaging the multitude of large and small muscles. Notice how the individual vertebrae in your spine separate and then rest back into each other as you breathe in and out. Notice how your ribs separate and then soften into each other on your in-breath and out-breath. Allow your head to gently rock with a "yes" and "no" motion at the top of your skull. Notice how each of these micro-movements cause a kinetic chain reaction of movement in the rest of your body. Breathe your awareness into your whole body at once, taking in this concert of micro-movements. This is the small dance.

Now, visualize yourself in a place where you do not feel comfortable to express your sexuality, where you feel your sexual self is not welcome. As you visualize this place, the environmental features and people there, notice how your small dance *may change its quality. Do the tiny adjustments become more abrupt or restrained? Do your vertebrae and ribs stay closer together? Notice the overall quality of this concert of micro-movements.*

Now release this visualization and invite in three full-body breaths. Softly allow your whole body to shake, allowing the emphasis to be on the dropping motions that fall in the direction gravity takes you like a "rag doll." Slowly bring your body back into stillness.

Next, visualize yourself in a place where you do feel comfortable expressing your sexuality. Notice the quality of your small dance *once this visualization is vivid in your imagination. Can you begin to deepen into your shifting balance, allowing the adjustments to fluidly sequence through from the base of your spine through the crown of your head as you lean from side to side, forward to back?*

> *You can also try this with a partner. As you focus your awareness on your somatic dance with gravity, invite a partner to place a hand on an agreed-upon location of your body (you can read ahead and include embodied touch here). Notice how your internal small dance shifts to accommodate this touch. Do you lean into the hand or away from it . . . or both? Once they remove their hand from your body, how does your dance find its independent balance once again? Try having them abruptly place and then abruptly remove their hand. Then have them slowly place and then slowly remove their hand. What are the differences in your dynamic alignment?*

Spatial Intent

This is the point where we cross over from exploring the way we inhabit our kinesphere to how we directly engage with or retract from the things and people within our environment. Spatial intent is how we communicate our needs and desires with our gaze, our words, or our movements—both large and small. Spatial intent can communicate interest through a subtle unipolar widening from our core through our left shoulder to lean into a sexual or romantic interest, an intense but smoldering gaze at the object of your attraction, or a full-bodied approach and embrace. It can also communicate disinterest through strongly averting your gaze or swiveling your head on your cervical spine away from someone with a unipolar narrowing (pulling the side body and shoulder into the midline) away from someone's body, or even a full-body palms flat and facing-forward "no." Spatial intent is the body's way of saying "I want that" or "I don't want this." It can also communicate "I am curious about that" while slowly moving in a direction. Spatial intent can also communicate "I'm not sure yet."

When I guide intimate partners in an exploration of spatial intent, I invite them to stand across the room from each other, take a few minutes to center themselves, and then connect with their partner at a distance. After they find something about their partner that they are attracted to, I invite them to follow the movement impulse to move closer to their partner in a way that expresses their inner intention and desire. I tell them that it is important that they not override any internal queue and move only at the pace of their desire or their interest. Some partners move in a straight line toward each other and, upon contact, fully embrace or start dancing. Other couples follow a slow and circuitous, almost teasing pathway toward each other. And still others follow a more start-and-stop rhythm to their spatial intent as they move toward what attracted them to their partner and then experience hesitance or fear and need to reset themselves before continuing on their path. One couple stayed right where they were across the room from each other and sent meaningful looks and sexy gestures toward each other. Their laughter and playful approach to the guidance sent a ripple of humorous response through me as we all laughed together. This couple's use of spatial intent is what Hackney (2002) refers to as the *psychological kinesphere*, the ability to extend beyond our ball of space with psychological qualities that can impact the tone of a whole room.

In non-monogamous relationships, intelligent spatial intent can support a grounded focus on one partner then another. When in intimate relationship with more than one person, the quality of attention given to each partner can at times feel distracted or split. According to Frankin Veaux and Eve Rickert, the authors of *More Than Two: A Practical Guide to Polyamory*, "there are more opinions being offered, more people's feelings to get hurt, more personalities to clash, more egos to bruise" (2014, pg. 14) in non-monogamous relationships. Far from an argument against polyamory, it is a call for more diligent and intentionally flexible awareness to support good communication skills and problem-solving. When supported by dynamic alignment, spatial intent can create a foundation for effectively oscillating attention as a multifocal awareness between more than two partners.

Spatial intent exploration allows us to learn about how our desire is expressed through movement and sound while honoring body sovereignty and embodied consent.

Erotic Bodyfulness Experiment With Spatial Intent

Stand or sit across from a sensorially delicious object (chocolate, a crystal, a painting, etc.) or a person (a lover, a friend, a sexy friend, etc.). Close your eyes and take three full-body breaths, allowing your body to adjust to accommodate more fullness of breath. With eyes still closed, see if your body can sense the object or the body of the other person. Find a place in your body that is communicating interest, curiosity, or pleasure. Breathe around this place and allow it to sequence out from the core of the sensation, down through your pelvic floor, and up through the crown of your head. Notice how your body adjusts its posture to accommodate this breath.

Now, open your eyes and connect visually with your object or with your person, either their gaze or taking them all in at once (panoramic focus is fine—direct gaze is not necessary here). How can you nonverbally sequence from the core of sensation out toward your object or person? Explore with sound, gaze, leaning movements, and moving toward. Allow your awareness to move toward your object or person directly from the core of sensation or desire.

Next, invite your spatial intent to soften and draw your felt sense into your back body. Rock back slightly onto your heels or the back of your

> *pelvic floor and breathe into your spine as you press into the space behind you with your back body. Rest.*
>
> *You can also explore with more than one person. Invite two people to sit with you. Close your eyes or soften your gaze and feel the presence of both people, oscillating your senses between them and back into your internal landscape. Now, open your eyes and oscillate your gaze from one person to the other, noticing how your internal landscape is impacted when you see one, then the other. What internal sensation changes between the two? Find your impulse for movement and sequence your reach from the core of your body to make connection with one person, rest and breathe, then pull yourself back into your center. Repeat this with the other person. What do you notice about the different sensations that arise with each person?*

Connect Your Back Body With Your Front Body

As a future-oriented, what-happens-next species, humans give the front of the body the most attention. The front of the body is what we see in the mirror and the part of us that faces others when we communicate. Yet the back body is a sensory-rich landscape full of information. As in the colloquial phrase "I'll back you up," the back body is also a place of resource and support.

The practice of directing your focus to awaken the awareness of your back body can have surprising results. During the 5Rhythms dance gatherings of Melissa Michaels, we often explore the awareness of the back body as a practice to develop a new perspective, build trust in our senses, and refine a skill to ground and regulate emotional activation. As we slowly walk backward in the room as a group, we may bump into one another. Instead of abruptly pulling away with an "oops!" reaction, Michaels invites us to pause, notice, and savor the connection before gently disconnecting and continuing our walk.

The back body can be engaged when placing your spine against a tree or sitting back-to-back with a friend or lover. In the yoga asana *Savasana*, the back body becomes the interface through which your bones and muscles release into the floor in total-body relaxation, supporting the integration of your yoga practice. Or lie with your belly on the floor, supporting the front body to calm the nervous system, and invite a friend or partner to place their hand on your back to feel your body further melt into the floor.

Why is this important to eroticism? Because when the front of your body is lurching forward with ungrounded arousal, the back body becomes an anchor to restore stability and honor body boundaries. Invite arousal energy to be anchored in the back body before sequencing your movement toward a partner. When the front body is tight and shielded and retreating from intimate contact, the back body becomes a resource to lean into the envelopment of safety. Lean into your back body until you feel a calming in your chest and belly and then resume contact when you feel ready. And when front-to-front contact with a partner feels too exposing, maybe when you are ready to reconnect after an argument, connecting your back bodies can be a pathway to grounded and gradual intimacy.

Also, when you equally expand your front and back body with your breath, your arousal energy can move more freely and pleasurably through the central corridor of your body.

Amplifying the Awareness of Your Back Body

Begin standing and invite three full breaths, emphasizing a long out-breath. As in the small dance practice earlier, connect your whole feet to the floor and center your hips above your feet while softening your knees. Lean forward slightly, feeling the forward direction of your front body. What draws your attention in front of you? Return to center and then slightly lean into your heels, breathing into your back body, expanding your spine, the back of your rib cage, and your sacrum (back of your pelvis). What is your back body aware of? Now, slowly let your back body guide you to walk backward to connect with what is behind you—a partner, a wall, a tree—and notice the impact on your inner somatic landscape as you make the first connection. Slowly, let your back body soften into the person or other surface. How much of you can you connect with the surface? Slowly press your spine, the back of your pelvis, and the back of your head with the surface behind you. If this is a person, can you feel the texture of their body, their breathing, their temperature? How does your body respond to this connection? Now, slowly begin to bring your body back to the midline, disengage from contact, and find balance over your feet and hips. How does your somatic landscape respond to the disconnection?

Depending on your body ability, you may also do this sitting. Connect your pelvic floor to the seat beneath you, your shoulders directly over your hips. Lean forward slightly and then return to center. Breathe into your back body, expanding your spine, the back of your rib cage, and your sacrum. Slowly, let your back body guide you to connect with the seat or person behind you. Notice the impact on your inner somatic landscape with the first connection. Allow your back body to soften into the person or surface behind you. Notice the quality of the surface, or the breathing and sensation of the person, behind you. Pause and notice what your back muscles and spine detect. Slowly, invite your posture back into balance, shoulders over hips, and notice what lingers from the contact.

Embodied Touch and Touching in Return

A warm hand on the cheek as we lean the side of our face into deeper contact. A slow glide over the lips with the fingers as our mouth opens, jaw and throat softening under the surprisingly erotic sensation. We have arrived at the moment where total body connectivity reaches out with consent for contact with our own body or the body of a lover.

Safe, loving, and pleasurable touch is the nutrient-dense soil of human relationship. Touch allows us to thrive in all ways and on all levels of the self. Even though infants may receive the necessities of food and shelter, those deprived of being touched or held do not thrive—instead they develop emotional, cognitive, and body integration deficiencies (Haradon, Bascom, Dragomir, & Scripcaru, 1994; Kim, Shin, & White-Traut, 2003). Meanwhile, infants who are given an abundance of safe and loving touch grow and flourish.

While adults do not need touch to objectively survive, they too need touch to continue to thrive. It is no accident that I often see clients who identify as low-touch attracting partners who are high-touch—their body craves it even if they often avoid it. Touch difference is a main point of contention that propels people to seek relationship counseling. Regardless of whether they are low-touch (rarely touch their partners and sometimes don't much enjoy being touched) or high-touch people (often touch their partners and really enjoy being touched), touch can be physically integrating and pleasurable. It can also communicate volumes about intention, desire, and mood by how it is offered and how it is received. In working with sexuality, it is of primary importance to apply total body connectivity to the realm of touch—consent for touch, intention of touch, and quality of touch—because it is most often the medium that comprises sex.

So often we haphazardly touch our own body and the bodies of others. We rush through a morning routine, roughly washing our skin or mindlessly applying lotion. We flop our hands onto our partner's body or grab their body parts in a slapdash fashion. Touch is expressed efficiently or in a habituated pattern. Taken for granted, the magnificence of skin-to-skin contact gets lost and we can feel confused and unsatisfied.

However, when applied as an intelligent tool in sex, touch can be alternately withheld and offered to heighten desire. Touch can be slowly, gradually intensified to spark arousal from a non-aroused, neutral state. Touch can be quick and intense, as it is in impact play, to snap us out of our heads and into an archetypal realm of dominance and submission. Touch can offer safety and love through long, deep, full-body holding. Skin-to-skin contact can regulate the nervous system, calming us from an activated state, and it can also amplify excitement and sensory attunement.

When we agree to conscious exchanges of pleasurable touch, we are engaging in a mindful and bodyful activity. Touch, therefore, is an opportunity for mind-body integration, relieving anxiety, stress, depression, and pain while increasing our personal effectiveness and improving our mood and outlook on life. In *Sensate Focus in Sex Therapy*, Weiner and Avery-Clark (2017) say that sex "is all about zeroing in on the sensations for yourself in the moment and without expectation for any particular response . . . to reconnect to the sensory roots of sexuality when you have become lost" (pg. 8). Touch literally aids us in feeling and connecting with ourselves and our experience of sexuality.

Touch and consent: Learning about the deep impact of the touch you offer and the touch you receive is a fundamental component of embodied sexuality and of the language of consent. Intimacy coach Betty Martin introduced the "Wheel of Consent" to support people in learning about the complexity of touch. Her wheel model contains four quadrants: *serve, take, allow,* and *accept.* Fundamentally, Martin's model is about awareness of our intention as we touch or are touched by a lover. When we make contact with a person's body, are we touching primarily for the other person's benefit (*serving*) or are we touching primarily for our benefit (*taking*)? And when our body is being touched by someone, are we *allowing* them to touch us more for their benefit or are we *accepting* the touch as something we desire? Usually, there is a combination of these intentions happening in the present moment, but keeping them in mind allows us to communicate more congruently—our internal intention aligning with the intention that we outwardly express. When combined with the total-body connectivity practices detailed earlier, both verbal and nonverbal expressions of consent become more pronounced.

Self-applied touch: Think about how you touch yourself. What type of contact do you make with your body when you are preparing for your day? Also, what type of contact do you offer yourself when you are happy or sad or angry? When you engage in solo sex or self-pleasure, how do you relate with your arousal anatomy (your genitals and other pleasure-inducing areas of the body)? How would you describe the quality of touch? Do you find that you take in food or other mind-body altering substances (this is another form of self-touch: via substance) in order to soothe yourself or give yourself pleasure? How we engage in touch with ourselves can give us a window into how we relate with our sexual body.

Touching yourself in intentional, loving, and pleasurable ways can facilitate embodied presence and cultivation of yourself as your own beloved as you love your sensual body and validate your own needs and desires. Dance/ movement therapist Kendra Seoane (2016) presents a model for self-applied touch as a healing and self-regulation tool—essentially a practice of learning to be the good-enough parent or partner to ourselves. By attuning with yourself—tracking your own sensations and moods and responding with loving and compassionate touch—you can "stabilize within an optimal state of arousal." This is the place where you can pendulate within your window of tolerance, the range in which you can integrate on emotional, physical, and cognitive levels. In other words, you can modulate your arousal with breath and movement to amplify a sense of presence without spilling out over your edges in reactive or dissociated ways. When the body tells us we are safe enough, our nervous system opens our senses wide, taking in more of the erotically relevant elements in our environment. Our social engagement system or Sexual Excitation System (SES), as sex educator Emily Nagoski calls it, is fully online. This is the place where we can enjoy being in a body and prioritize our own pleasure while maintaining a respectful relationship with a partner.

Loving and sensual self-applied touch is an essential component of having an embodied relationship with ourselves. Through our physical relating with and honoring of ourselves, we can learn about what we find pleasurable without the performance anxiety that can occur with a partner. We are more likely to speak up and advocate for our pleasure and our boundaries. We can hold our own heart and give love to our own arousal anatomy. Practice intentionally applying lotion to your skin and massaging your muscles. Practice holding yourself or your heart when you are happy or when you are sad. Slow down and let your touch be loving and pleasurable toward yourself.

Erotic Bodyfulness Experiment With Embodied Self-Applied Touch

Sit or stand in a comfortable position. If you choose to sit, tilt the top of your pelvis forward slightly to connect your pelvic floor with your seat beneath you and let the crown of your head guide your spine upward to lengthen. If you are standing, soften your knees and lengthen your tailbone toward the ground as the crown of your head guides your spine to lengthen toward the ceiling. Breathe three full breaths while adjusting your body as needed to make room for more breath.

With only your body awareness (no physical touch just yet), locate the center of your chest. Feel your breath expanding the space around your heart. Starting directly from this place at the middle of your chest, let your awareness travel from around your heart, through your shoulder, all the way down your arm, and into the palm of your hand. Let this sequencing of awareness then extend with your movement as you slowly raise your hand to connect your full palm and fingers with the front of your chest. Notice how your hand settles into place over your chest. Breathe and soften your shoulders. What happens to the sensation in your chest as you make contact?

Keeping your hand on your chest, locate your belly or womb space with your awareness. Breathe and expand your belly and pelvic floor.

Notice the sensations here and begin to sequence your awareness from your belly/womb, up through your chest, and through your other shoulder, arm, and hand. Now let your movement sequence with your awareness as you slowly place your other hand on your belly. Breathe and soften your shoulders, jaw, and flower open your pelvic floor. Notice how the internal landscape of your belly responds to this contact as your hand settles onto the curvature of your lower body.

Now with both hands on your body, what do you want your hands to communicate to your body? You get to choose. "You are beautiful." "You are worthy of pleasure."

You can repeat this activity while sequencing your movement to hold or cup your face, your hips, or your genitals, all while breathing, softening, and inviting pleasure.

Touch between you and a partner: Giving and receiving. Reciprocity. Mutual pleasure. Exchanging pleasurable touch with a lover or play partner can be a delightful gateway into the altered state of arousal and into deeper connection. Neuroscientist Stephen Porges describes the process of touch: relational safety allows for closer proximity, followed by touch, which leads to deeper bonding—not just commitment, but a felt sense of being bonded with another human. This is an important distinction. We don't always have sex with a partner from a place of feeling safe or a place of interest or pleasure. Like walking with a wounded leg, we have sex while protecting our softer, more vulnerable parts, thereby disengaging contact from a total body connection with ourselves. When we do it for them, or we feel they are doing it for us, our experiences are left sorely wanting.

On the other hand, practicing embodied touch with a partner gives us an opportunity to connect with the veracity of our wanting—we move forward with contact as our body tells us we are truly open to touching and being touched. We connect with the core of our body or a pleasurable sensation and allow our reach for contact to be sourced directly from this origin place with the support of our breath and spatial intent. When the direction of the desired movement takes us away from contact, that is our truth telling us we want to slow down, change position, or stop. When our partner is supportive of our gesture away from them, which they communicate with slowing down, a connected gaze, or checking in, they are saying to you, "Thank you for telling me that." They are validating the truth of the body. This validation underscores the safety of the connection and softens the nervous system, and perhaps then the pleasurable exchange can resume.

Embodied offer of touch: Touch can be offered by any part of the body, including the fingers and hands, and it can be received by any part of the body—as long as it is agreed upon or requested by your partner(s). Whether touch is initiated by the hands, a cheek, a side body or back body, or the genitals, touch originates from the point of first desire, inch by inch, with the support of breath through to the place of contact. As you offer your touch, engage the erotic bodyfulness practice to slow your awareness and continue to link up with the present moment.

Erotic Bodyfulness Experiment of Offering Touch

Read this passage aloud with your play partner before beginning. Let your partner tell you what area of their body where they would enjoy feeling contact during this experiment. Determine a time frame for the contact. I recommend 15 to 20 minutes to start because this is the general length of time that the nervous system takes to feel a shift, moving from the Sexual Inhibition System (SIS) to the Sexual Excitation System (SES).

Sit in a comfortable position, pelvic floor connected with your seat beneath you. Invite three full breaths and do a scan of your somatic landscape. Find one or two sensations as anchors. Now, see your partner, either with your eyes or with your environmental awareness senses. What about your play partner is interesting or attractive to you? As you see your partner, tune into your own body and scan your somatic landscape for a feeling of pleasure, interest, desire, or curiosity. Once you find the source of desire or interest within the landscape of the body, fill this land-mark with breath. As we explored earlier, the breath begins the outward movement toward what we desire. With the consent of your partner (a verbal "yes" or a bodily "yes" of opening, softening, and expanding toward you), allow the breath to carry the sensation from the origin point to the surface of your body. Pressing and anchoring down the lower body and pelvic floor (dynamic alignment), let your breath continue to carry your movement sequence into the reach toward the body of your partner with your cheek, hands, or other part of the body. Once contact is made, begin in stillness, savoring the moment of skin on skin. Too often, initial contact gives way to a frenzy of touch. This can initiate a disconnection from our present moment awareness and a disconnection from our partner and their experience. Once you have savored the contact and yielded (active rest) into the present moment, then slowly begin exploring your partner's body in the area they have given consent. As touch progresses, continue to oscillate your awareness between different areas of your body and between you and your partner. When you hear or feel a request to slow down or stop (when you see or feel a physical retraction, stillness, or lack of deep breath in your partner), slow your movement and check in with your partner. Explore together what is needed to find that softening and fullness of breath before continuing.

As your touch session comes to a close, bring your hands back to stillness on your partner's body. Breathe and settle your awareness into your pelvic floor and back body. Press your connected body part into your play partner once more and then slowly draw yourself back to your center, gently removing contact and fully reconnecting with yourself.

Share with your partner your experience of this and invite them to share their experience as well. Share with each other what qualities of touch felt enjoyable.

Embodied receiving of touch: When we receive touch from ourselves or from a lover, we are not simply passive recipients or static objects. No matter what our response is to being touched—whether we get butterflies, soften, retract, or dissociate—we are always impacted. As previously said, touch is an opportunity to feel ourselves, to understand our desires and our boundaries, and to be an active participant in relationship. With the foundation of total body connectivity, we can refine our phenomenological felt sense and outward expression of pleasure. This can deepen our enjoyment of contact as well as clearly communicate to a partner whether we enjoy the touch they offer.

As you receive touch that feels good to you, invite in a full breath and reach your senses out toward the place of contact. Your full breath expands the boundary of your body, increasing surface area to be touched and communicating a feeling of pleasure. Using your breath and subtle body movement toward contact, you can literally *touch your partner back* through the bipolar or unipolar widening of your shape flow. When this expansion of your body toward contact feels like a "yes," try verbally communicating "yes" or "that feels good." Do those words feel congruent to you? In order to honor consent in sex, that moment-to-moment check-in and communication of the physical and verbal "yes" is essential. Remember, a verbal "yes" can be the actual word, or a sigh, or even a soft "mmm-hmmm" as you expand and lean further into contact.

Erotic Bodyfulness Experiment With Embodied Receiving

You can practice embodied receiving with self-applied touch, an object like a flower, and a play partner.

Sit in a comfortable position, connecting your pelvic floor with the seat beneath you, and invite in three full breaths to feel the present moment. Scan your somatic landscape for initial sensation and adjust or stretch your body to make space for more breath. Bring your own hand into contact with a place on your body (for example, over your heart, belly, or genitals). Notice the somatic impact of this contact, taking an inventory of inner sensations, temperature, micro-movements, and sense of volume. Now, expand your breath toward the area of contact and follow the expansion from your breath to subtly lean or press your body into the contact. After you expand on the in-breath, allow your body to soften into your seat on the out-breath, and then invite the next in-breath into your back body (spine, back muscles, sacrum). On your next in-breath, expand your breath to carry your skin closer to the place of contact again. Activate your interoceptive senses (which detect internal activity) to notice how your body is impacted by this contact.

Next, with your partner, let them know what area of your body you would like to receive touch. Do a body scan of your internal landscape to get a baseline of your sensations. Encourage your partner to begin with stillness as they place their hand on your body. Invite your in-breath to connect your pelvic floor with your seat more deeply and allow your out-breath to engage a moment of active rest. Can you find a place of warmth, tingling, or another sense of pleasure within your body or at the skin level? If you find this place, surround it with breath. Then let your breath guide your awareness from the origin point of sensation toward the place of contact, while staying aware of the space around you. Subtly press into contact, letting your widening body guide your skin to touch your partner back. Notice how your inner landscape is impacted by this gesture of feeling contact deeply and touching your partner with your body. Notice the impact on your breath, sensation, and spatial intent once contact is initiated. What is your next movement impulse?

From the Inside Out

By developing the skill of full-effort erotic expressiveness—combining breath support with sequencing movement, dynamic alignment, spatial intent, and embodied touch—you can use your body knowledge to intelligently engage in and navigate sexual connections. Total-body connectivity is a lived expression of personal empowerment. When we connect with personal power, we can impact the world in which we are embedded—relationships, creative projects, even the natural environments we steward. This slow (in awareness, not necessarily movement) and bodyful process is the bedrock upon which we dismantle assumptions and judgments about our sexual bodies to rebuild anew from the truth of the moment-to-moment dance of bodies. Those who erotically express themselves with clear effort move through the world, from the inside out, with truth and clarity.

8

YOUR EROTIC MAP

Mapping the Sexual Self

Within you is a sexuality constellation, a group of moments that form a recognizable pattern. This pattern is a map for you as you journey to work intelligently with your erotic self in order to better inform your intimate relationships. While individual sexuality is vast, your own experience of eroticism is much more specific—the realm of the erotic is composed of the core elements that activate and awaken your sexuality, the obstacles and challenges that compel your latent energy, and the primordial shadow that pulls on you from beneath your conscious awareness. Because of the deeply internal and complex nature of sexuality, this constellation, this map of erotic factors, is often difficult to fully grasp in any usable detail without a structure. To further complicate matters, our culture's adolescent sexuality keeps many of us stuck in a limited or fearful perspective on the erotic. We muck about in the shallow murkiness of sexuality, waiting to be inspired, for something to happen "naturally," for a good. Long. Time.

The erotic mapping process presented in this chapter will show you a mirror of your experience, clearing the murkiness while still making space for your mystery to continue to unfold over time. This mapping allows you to become the captain of your vessel—the clouds clear and you may now steer from atop the helm with visible constellations of stars as your guide. This map of the sexual self is unique to you. It is based on your experiences and family lineage, and, while it evolves over time, the underlying currents are often consistent. And it is this collection of the points of interest for *you* that encompass how your erotic life is formed and how it is expressed.

This chapter presents the process of crafting your erotic map from the information that you have gathered about yourself in prior chapters and directly from the somatic experience of your sexuality landscape. The personal

DOI: 10.4324/9780429297236-9

information that you have assembled can now be organized within the three main areas of your erotic map, as well as in the spaces where the realms intersect. The three main areas of the map highlight where one is *masterful*, reveals where one experiences *challenge*, and sheds light on the *shadow* realm of sexuality. As you oscillate between the somatic experience of your body landscape and the map that you craft visually onto paper, you are invited to revel when ecstasy is found and identify where the hard work must be done. This presents you with an embodied pathway to move more freely between the realms and, therefore, to move more freely through your intimate and creative life.

Within the interconnected realms of the erotic map we find how we relate to ourselves, how we relate to others, what invites our desire to surface, and what pushes our desire and arousal underground. The spaces of overlap between these three areas reveal the information that is needed to *move* us—physically, emotionally, and mentally—from unconscious reaction toward conscious and effective response. This information can give you an overall sense of self-understanding, a wider range of acceptance for yourself and your partner(s), and a sense of evolving personal empowerment. In your map you may find resource and refuge, as well as difficulty and uncertainty. We need both support and challenge to grow and refine our intimate complexity. We need to be empowered individuals who creatively participate in relationships and in the social sphere. When we are unaware of the aspects of the erotic self, we can unconsciously (and sometimes negatively) impact others and we will have increased difficulty navigating our social-sexual environments.

Your sociocultural context, the proverbial waters that surround your erotic map, saturate your sexual mastery as well as your shadows with fertile and demanding currents. This map lives in the push-pull as well as the resonance with your family and the concentric layers of your life that inform your erotic self. We are set up to accept certain parts of our sexuality as well as deny or feel shame for other parts of our sexuality. Embodying our individual expressions of sexuality often feels as though we are swimming upstream, against the strong current. Overcoming this challenge is the bread and butter of people-making. Your erotic map will guide you to the route that will carry you through the eddies and raging rapids of these often treacherous sociocultural waters.

As erotic maps shift and change over the life span, I recommend that my clients create their maps before and after life transitions (like becoming a parent or committing to a partnership) or after transitioning through a developmental milestone, and over the course of our work together in order to recognize the evolution of their sexual self.

When our erotic map collides and interweaves with the erotic map of a partner or lover, a third erotic map is created. The interweaving of erotic maps will be covered in Chapter 9.

The Erotic Mapping Process

The process of creating an erotic map involves a visualization process and an embodied movement process. This allows the erotic map to be both image based and somatic based, thus integrating the whole self. With image, we engage the imagination of the mind and with somatic movement, we activate expression in real time. Aphorist Mason Cooley said, "Fantasy mirrors desire. Imagination reshapes it." For the visualization component, you can create your map on a whiteboard, as a collage, a painting, etc.—whatever method helps you document and organize your constellation points in a form that is accessible and pleasing to your senses. The erotic map is accompanied by the movement explorations described in Chapter 7. The embodied movement process is a movement sequence designed to both generate erotic energy and contain it.

The information found within the three main points of interest of an erotic map—masterful, challenge, and shadow—include the lessons I have been sharing in each chapter so far: erotic gateways (what ignites desire and turns you on and what creates revulsion and turns you off), experience of sexual response cycle (experience of desire, arousal, flow space, peak experiences, and integration), forms of sexual expression through voice/movement/gesture, and your experience as a sexual being in your sociocultural location. By exploring each of these areas, we consider your relationship to your body, your relationship to your lineage where potential shadow material dwells, impactful social messages, and your relationship to power dynamics.

We will use the skill of erotic bodyfulness at each point of interest on the erotic map to study your somatic landscape and larger expressive movements that present themselves in your mastery, challenge, and shadow areas. One movement sequence will be crafted and clarified for each realm and then connected through a loose choreography that bridges all three areas. This becomes the movement process of your map to learn about your sexual expression as well as a way of directing you to your resilience.

Now, let's explore the basic erotic map one component at a time.

The Realm of Full-Effort Resource: Mastery and Ease

While you can begin to explore your erotic map from anywhere on the basic map (seen in Figure 8.1), I often have my clients start in the realm of mastery and easeful effort. Somatic therapist Ruby Gibson (2008) begins the process of Somatic Archaeology with her clients by asking "what is right with you?" (pg. 13). Gibson encourages those doing healing work to "put much more emphasis on your delight than on your drama" (pg. 14). As discussed earlier, exploring the sexual self can be a rough and muddy road, so beginning where

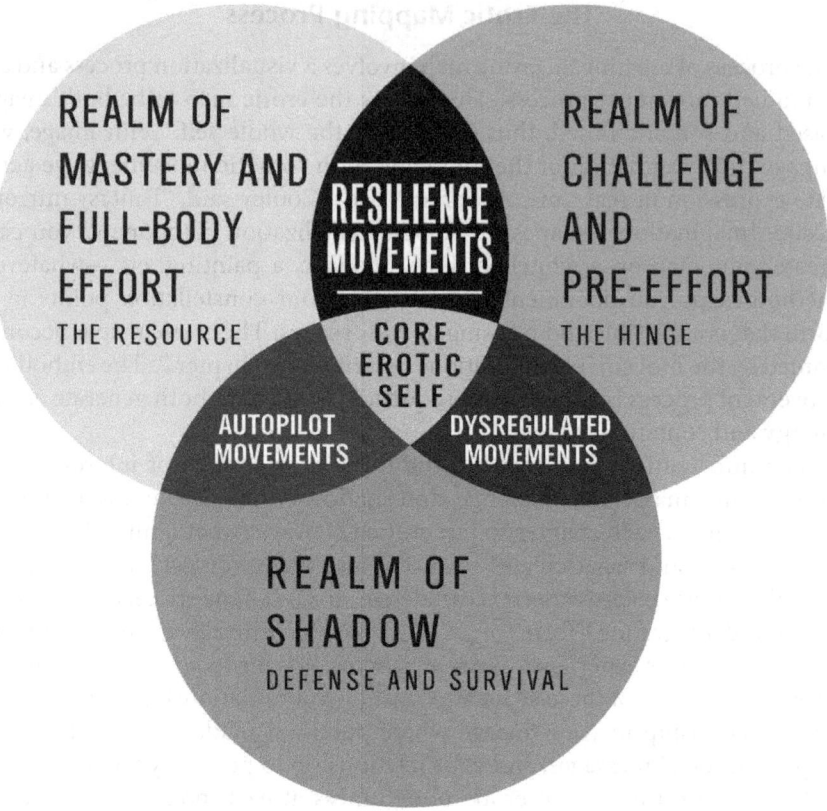

Figure 8.1 Basic Erotic Map by Melissa Walker, MA, LPC, CST, R-DMT

we find resource can not only ease tensions, but also create a solid anchor to return to when the sky gets cloudy on your adventure.

This mastery realm is where your sexual energy has been allowed and invited to flow freely. These are the open doorways that you are uninhibited to walk through or the doorways you have worked hard to create for yourself. This realm of mastery is possible because sexual energy always finds a way through the body armor to expression, even when one has experienced great cultural, familial, or social pressure to inhibit expression or has experienced violation. Creative music and art expression among oppressed and marginalized people is a great example of how this realm is formed. When we are constricted and minimized in our lives, sexual energy still flows through the cracks that are formed under pressure, creating the most achingly beautiful artifacts of human culture. These artifacts then become a refuge and a resource.

In Chapter 7, "Erotic on the Outside," we talked about full-effort movement as an expression of mastery and easefulness, as the sort of embodied experience that is marked by feeling safe enough and excited enough to enjoy the feeling of being in a body. Full-effort movement expresses one's ability to "effectively cope with environmental challenges" (Kestenberg-Amighi, Loman, & Sossin, 2018, pg. 89). This realm, therefore, is the bodyful experience of what dancer, physical therapist, and dance therapy trailblazer Irmgard Bartenieff called *Total Body Connectivity*, where we experience "a lively interplay of internal connectivity with outer expressivity" (Hackney, 2002, pg. 34) enriching our life. Within the realm of full effort, pleasure is more easily accessible; body movement is a little bigger with more free-flow, strong, or direct qualities; and the breath is full and deep. When I explore this realm with my clients, it is common for them to name activities like their favorite workout, pastime, or hobby, or a cherished vacation spot. They name sexual play where they easily access pleasure, orgasm, or partner connection. This is most often accompanied by a somatic experience of feeling relaxed, warm, tingly, in the flow, empowered, or confident. In other words, they experience more free-flow movement instead of constricted and bound flow. This is not the issue that you are grappling with which caused you to pick up this book— the realm of full effort is the place of hope and resilience that knows you can work through challenge and adversity. We may arrive at experiences of full effort in our eroticism by chance or create them ourselves to balance out the places where shadow has touched our lives.

As I explore this realm with Rachael, her whole face lights up as she describes what she loves to do. Costuming, special-effects makeup, and the theater—these are the things that open her to the experience of embodied excitement and confidence. Once she was adorned in her creations and stepping onstage for her performance, Rachael feels effortlessly sexy and expansive. This is a far cry from her experience of middle school where she was bullied for her appearance—a full-figured and dark-skinned Latina in a mostly white suburban school. The bullying could have been a brick wall to her erotic expression, yet through creative costuming and acting, Rachael's sexual energy found a way to flow around the rocks in the river.

Take also my client Russ, a white, middle-aged market analyst who is troubled by his increasing difficulty with erections. While exploring his area of mastery, he describes how much he loves to sing, especially while being witnessed by other people. In my office, I have him describe the experience of singing karaoke (one of his favorite hobbies) while standing to free up any movement impulses that emerge during the somatic exploration. As he closed his eyes and described standing onstage while belting out "I Was Made for Loving You" by KISS, I saw his knees bend slightly and the crown of his head reach for the ceiling. His face widened into a smile and his breathing dropped into his belly. He described the openness and rays of heat from his solar plexus up through his chest and out through his shoulders. When I invited him to sink into his feet and rise up with the heat rays through his shoulders in one continuous sweeping and spreading motion, his breath deepened further and his face flushed with color. He laughed and said, "Man, this feels so good. I could just take up the whole room!" As we further explored his experience, we discovered that his enjoyment of singing karaoke was marked by a full-body engagement and the building rhythm of the song to a crescendo, followed by a thunderous finish before stillness set in and the anticipation of the next song began to build again.

This rhythm—what we dance therapists call *surging and birthing* (Kestenberg-Amighi, Loman, & Sossin, 2018, pg. 48)—is a generative life rhythm found in many creative processes. At first, the more indulging (mobilizing and merging) swaying rhythm—a developmental rhythm characterized by relaxation and nurturing sensations—builds within us to the fighting (intense and differentiating) rhythm of surging and birthing. It harnesses the intensity of creation by challenging our abilities in the pressurized movement of creation. This is often described as an ecstatic feeling. Interestingly, surging and birthing is also the rhythm of orgasm. This was a place of resource and revitalization for my client.

As you read this, you may be thinking that your experience of resource may be different than Russ's sweet spot. Your masterful, resourced sexuality may feel more like the pleasurable experience of the snapping/biting rhythm indicative of activities like kickboxing or impact play for kinksters. Or you may really enjoy the sucking or swaying rhythm of languishing in a hammock on a warm day or during slow lovemaking sessions. Or you may prefer the twisting rhythms that appear in flirtation and delay-of-pleasure practices. Let's explore how your sexuality mastery shows up for you.

Erotic Bodyfulness Exploration

Find Your Mastery: The "Resource"

On your erotic map, the realm of mastery is the upper left circle of the three-circle Venn diagram in Figure 8.1. This is the realm of resource—the aspects of your sexuality that you can rely on and return to when you want to de-stress, fill your bucket, and generally feel good. Identify where you feel erotically masterful, easeful, relaxed, or excited. Explore the landscape of your sexuality: perhaps you feel mastery in an aspect of your gender expression, your sex life, your relationships, your pleasurable hobbies, or your connection with your body. What aspects of these various realms feel like a pleasurable or erotic resource?

Take a few moments to visualize where you feel masterful and easeful in your sexuality. What really peaks your attention and pleasure? What do you rely on to get into a better mood? Getting the full benefit of this

realm involves an erotic bodyfulness exploration. As you turn your aware-
ness to the experience of your body, oscillating your attention between the
awareness of your mind and the awareness of the landscape of your body,
notice the qualities of sensation that arise. Notice your muscle tension or
openness, temperature, breath quality, and micro- or macro-movements.
Repeat any movement that arises here until your movement feels clear
and repeatable, full of breath support, and extending from the core of
your body to the endpoints of your fingers, toes, crown of the head, and
tailbone.

In your journal, record this internal somatic awareness and movements
using descriptive, sensory language. We will return to this realm after vis-
iting the challenge and shadow areas.

The Realm of Challenge: Interest and Obstacle

The realm of challenge on your erotic map is where you find both excitement
and nervousness, curiosity and uncertainty, expression combined with suppression. This is the realm that contains the aspects of sexuality that most
often inspire people to seek professional therapeutic support. This is also the
realm where we find attraction to sociocultural taboos; in taboo, interest and
pleasure are combined with discomfort in the form of shame or hesitancy.
This combination can cause a fixation on the taboo, reducing our ability to
consciously engage with the deeper meaning underneath the attraction to
the taboo or to engage in satisfying and fulfilling relationships while still
honoring our own desires. It is important to note that what is taboo for some
is fully acceptable for others. One person could be raised in a family or culture that supports public displays of affection while another person could
be raised with the belief that affection in front of others is exhibitionist and
inappropriate. In intimate or committed relationship, this clash of accept-
ability can produce misunderstanding and conflict. We value relationships
so much that we will often suppress a part of ourselves that we feel doesn't fit
within our connection with others. We do this to maintain what my mentor,
Leah D'Abate, refers to as the "love and sanctuary of our relationships." We
would rather withhold a need and desire than "rock the boat" and risk losing
our closeness. Challenge—the grist for the mill—comes from attempting to
balance which of our needs we can express while maintaining relationships.

Challenge is also present when sexuality and connection to pleasure are
impacted by chronic illness, an overworked or exhausting schedule, or relationship difficulties. Physical or emotional pain can impede our pleasurable
connection with our body by activating a bound-flow response in the nervous system—we tighten the muscle and soft tissue structures around areas
of pain. This causes us to be more tuned into the noxious elements within us

and within our environments. Do you notice that, while you desire intimacy and space for pleasure, you cannot access connection with your body or your partner because you are so stressed from work, parenting, or other weights on your shoulders? These types of stressors leave us stuck in our minds, distracted and exhausted.

While an aspect of your sexuality may be an embodied resource in one context, this same aspect may feel like a challenge in other areas. My client Liz could find herself solidly within her full expression of sexuality or deep in shadow in relationship to her sensual body. As a mixed-race woman, half white and half black, Liz was all too familiar with the experience of her body code-switching between worlds. "When I travel alone to the coast, I really enjoy floating in the ocean. It's the most sensual pleasure in the world. But when I travel with my friends, I start to feel self-conscious about my body. They always comment on dieting or how their clothes fit. They don't say it to me directly, but I can feel their criticism in my direction too. I can't enjoy being in my body, let alone relax in the waves. It triggers my self-consciousness and I start to criticize myself." This is challenge. For Liz, her challenge of enjoying the sensuality of her body near the ocean is a hinge. In one situation, being in her body is the best experience in the world, but it can also bend toward her shadow, depending on how she is being witnessed and who is witnessing her.

The gift is that the challenge *can* hinge toward masterful instead of dropping into the reactions and reactivity of the shadow realm. As human mammals, we truly live for facing challenge and adversity and are fortified by the experience of mobilizing in the face of obstacles. Under the right conditions, our bodies can thrive from exposure to stress. For example, Dialectical Behavior Therapy, a psychotherapeutic modality aimed at alleviating some of the most difficult mood disorders, proposes TIPP skills (temperature change, increased heart rate, paced breathing, and progressive relaxation) to halt panic attacks and jolt the body out of a depressive episode. The first component, temperature change, encourages submerging your face in ice-cold water to reset the nervous system. Activating the body's stress response on a sensory level provides relief. This may seem counterintuitive, but avoiding discomfort pushes our difficult emotions deeper into the shadow where they can truly run amok and lower our ability to tolerate emotional distress. However, when we face discomfort head-on with our personal resources at the ready, our emotional immune system is boosted and fortified.

When we use personal resourcing skills to maintain mobility within our window of tolerance, the stress created by challenge can fuel personal growth, which then supports the development of resilience. The experience of resilience—a confidence in our ability to face adversity and also bounce back after adversity—shows up on the physiological level as an adaptable *tone* in the vagus nerve of our central nervous system. The vagus nerve is the central corridor of the central nervous system, connecting primary body systems such as the lungs and digestion with the somatic nervous system of muscles and tissues, allowing the body to mitigate the stress response. If you have a *hypertonic* vagal response, you find that you overreact to stress and have a difficult time calming down after a stressful event. If you have a *hypotonic* vagal response, you may experience being frozen or dissociated, or may even faint, in response to stress. Resilience is the sweet spot in between where your nervous system has a flexible quality in response to stress.

Within the realm of challenge on the erotic map, you are invited to use erotic bodyfulness skills to work with the challenge and grow your resilient vagal tone. This resilience gives us the strength and wisdom to call ourselves back from the edge of the abyss and explore what may be confusing or difficult with an awake and resilient set of personal skills.

Finding Your Challenge: The "Hinge"

In order to identify your core challenges in sexuality, you can explore the aspects of self where you feel both turned on and constricted, curious and anxious, interested yet hesitant. Even though part of you wants to look away, you find yourself compelled. For example, you may often find yourself close to genital orgasm, yet you cannot release to the full expression of bodily ecstasy. Or you may be curious about anal play (or other sexual behavior) but notice self-judgments crowding your mind when you fantasize about it. Or you may long to be more fluid in your gender, yet do not yet feel safe enough to embody this in public. A challenge can also be something where you feel nourished by your sexuality in one context while shameful or embarrassed about it in a different context.

Take a few moments to close your eyes and scan the map of your sexuality. Where do you currently feel challenged? As you visualize the aspects of your sexuality—sexual activities, gender, orientation—notice the experience of your whole self. Within the landscape of your body, notice the distinctive somatic characteristics of challenge: opening and warmth in one area of your body with constriction or shakiness and discomfort in another area—two seemingly opposing experiences happening simultaneously. Invite breath and soften your muscular structure around these seemingly conflicting areas. Give your muscles the permission to do the movement they need to so that you get a better sense of your somatic experience.

Within your mind, notice the thoughts that accompany your challenge— the judgments, assumptions, self-criticism, and invalidations, as well as the thoughts hinging toward understanding and compassion. Notice the complexity of emotion that arises. What are the involuntary or "shadow"

> *(not obvious or intentional) movements that automatically happen as you visualize your challenge—facial expressions, movements in your limbs, movement sensations beneath your skin. What happens in your pelvis? Your stomach, your chest area, your throat? Do you have awareness of your back body? Do you find yourself leaning forward or backward and off-balance from your central alignment? Allow the movements that arise to become exaggerated as you explore the sensations that build. Repeat the movements that arise until there is more clarity in the trajectory and quality of your articulation.*
>
> *Record in your journal what you are aware of within the realm of challenge on your erotic map. Using descriptive and sensory language, record your somatic experience and the movement qualities that arose. Does this movement sequence and sensory experience feel familiar from another area of your life? Consider personal, work, and family realms.*

The Realm of Shadow: Opening Pandora's Box

As was discussed in Chapter 3, the realm of shadow holds our blind spots—the beliefs, values, behaviors, and experiences of which we are unaware or which we intentionally or unintentionally suppress. Like the bubbles on the surface of the "Bog of Eternal Stench" in Jim Henson's *Labyrinth*, we become aware of our shadow when it erupts, like fetid bubbles to the surface. It becomes evident that my clients have passed into the shadow realm when I hear them say things like, "No one finds me sexy," "I'm not worth it," or "Everyone leaves me." Suddenly, the air has been sucked out of the room; they narrow toward their midline and freeze or they lash out in sudden anger. Like sinkholes, these absolute statements are clothed in dark and pervasive assumptions. They suck the very life from Eros, the love nature of the erotic. This is the place where simply being in our skin can be unbearable. We are entrenched in discomfort and helplessness.

It is not just the unsavory experiences or parts of ourselves that are found here. We also find our greatest gifts and characteristics within the realm of shadow—the parts of our personality and expression that we hide because it is too vulnerable to share them with the world. These are the parts of ourselves that we buried in order to be accepted by family or friends. Yet often the parts of self that we quarantine for safety are our most beautiful and inspiring features.

I know that this can all sound dark and scary. Yet it is normal to have shadows. *We all have them* and we always will. And while you may find yourself wanting to skip this section because of the discomfort, the secret to healing and integrating your sexuality resides in forming a relationship with your shadows, slowly, and with support. Fear of the shadow realm can be assuaged by honing our skills to relate with and uncover the deeper meaning hidden in our own Pandora's box. When we dare to look into that box, while anchored in resource, we find that sexual shadows are also the big obstacles that can fuel deep personal growth and cultivate our power.

It was this fuel that is uncovered in my work with Rachael. As we explore the realm of shadow, I notice that her torso becomes very still, her breathing almost imperceptible, and her mouth held closed in a tight line, as she recalls being bullied for her hair and skin color as a young Latinx teenager in a mostly white suburban school. As she shrinks toward the midline of her body, I invite her bound muscles to tell Rachael how they were trying to take care of her by pulling tight to her midline. "If I am smaller, I won't be seen. Being seen is dangerous. It's not safe."

I then invite Rachael to breathe into the back of her pelvis, pressing into the cushions behind her. After a few full in-breaths and out-breaths, I see her shoulders soften apart toward her hips and her mouth soften at the corners. I encourage her access the movement bridge toward her masterful gesture, the resource we discovered when she is costumed and acting onstage. Gradually, her breath sweeps her arms up to arc overhead like a great sun. She repeats this sweeping and arcing gesture several times. I can see her sequencing this movement directly from her core to the furthest reaches of her endpoints. With each repetition, she becomes more full, clear, and expansive. Her eyes opened and clarity returned as we again connected our gaze. "Remember that scene in *Lord of the Rings* where Frodo can't remember the taste of strawberries?" she asked me. "I was almost there." The realm of shadow could pull her under, into the darkness like the one created by Sauron in the *Lord of the Rings* trilogy. Yet, by anchoring herself in the erotic resource with breath and clear movement, Rachael could also be the Samwise character, the one who calls her back into the light, back to the taste of summer strawberries.

By refining our ability to access self-compassion and the resilience that most assuredly lives within us all, we can bridge ourselves back into conscious connection, carrying the gems from the dark below in our grateful hands.

Explore Your Shadow

Here is your opportunity to lift the lid of your box of shadows. Before you begin, remember the masterful resource movement that you recorded earlier. The breath quality and movement of the realm of resource will be a place to return to when the pull of the shadow becomes too much. Remember, if we plunge too deeply, too fast, we miss the hidden landmarks by blowing past them and we just replay an old and unconscious pathway of coping. Take a moment now to revisit the visualization and corresponding movement of your resilient sexuality.

Now, soften your gaze and visualize the aspects of your sexuality where you feel discomfort or darkness. What are the criticisms of yourself or your partner(s) that you notice your mind telling you? What are the memories or dreams that you actively avoid remembering? What are the difficult stories of your past that you tell without emotion or with overwhelming emotion? What are the historical stories told to you about your lineage by your older family members? Notice what happens in your inner somatic landscape—the sensations, temperature, and involuntary movements. Do you notice constriction, rigidity, or numbness? Is your breathing shallow and fast, or frozen in a confined area of the body? Notice the direction the movement is taking you and, for just a moment, exaggerate the movement already happening in your body.

Make a few notes in your journal using sensory and descriptive words. Also record the criticisms and judgments that arise.

Return to resource: Allow yourself a full, long out-breath and return to the visualization of your mastery resource. You may notice difficult emotions now filling your chest and jaw—anger, sadness, anxiousness, grief. Notice if there are tears and support their release with your out-breath and softening of jaw and shoulders. A strong out-breath, soft downward shaking motion of your whole body, and breathing into your back body may release tears, which are instrumental in helping emotions move, like a clog being flushed from a pipe. Take a drink of water, go for a walk outside, or engage in a desired activity. Ask for a long hug from a trusted loved one. If you are still feeling tightness in your body, meet the intensity in your muscles with push-ups or a run. If you are feeling exhausted, engage in something restorative like a cup of tea, a massage, or sleep. Visiting the shadow is not about re-traumatizing or ruminating in the negative. Instead, taking a walk through the dark is about gaining wisdom and integrating parts of you that previously were left alone in the shadows. This requires intentional self-care afterward, so don't skimp on the time you take to care for your body and heart. It is vital to integration that you do so!

The Space Between: Overlapping Gateways

Our erotic resources, challenges, and shadows do not exist as islands living an isolated existence. Try as we might, we cannot forever stay in the relaxed bliss of doing something we love or interacting with the most exciting and riveting challenges. Difficult challenges will inevitably present themselves. Shadows surface in the most inconvenient, yet poignant, moments. Instead of existing separately, the spaces between the realms are the gateways that contain important information about how we transition from one state to another. When we face an erotic obstacle, how do we resource enough to stay in the present moment? When we get stuck in a narrow experience of unsatisfying pleasure, how do we again broaden our erotic repertoire to incorporate other, more satisfying, sources of pleasure? When we get triggered and exit ourselves, how do we come back? The dynamic movement offered by these transition spaces allows for the development of that resilient vagal tone through action and mobilization through the stuck places. Through the new movement sequences, you will develop mastery and have empowered choice. This is what defines the dynamic potential of being in a body.

Now that you have visited each of the three main realms with corresponding somatic awareness and movements, you can discover for yourself the power of intentional action as you express through movement around your erotic map. The overlapped areas show you how your resources are born from or offer reprieve from your shadows and how your challenges can cause you to dysregulate into shadow or integrate into resource. It is within these in-between gateways that we are shown what the body psychotherapy modality of Hakomi calls *organicity*—our continual, psychobiological proclivity for growth and change.

Resilience: Between the Mastery and Challenge Realms

The gateway between your mastery realm—the realm of sexuality resource— and your challenge realm—the "hinge"—is an oasis of intelligent resilience. Resilience is our ability to recover from difficulty, to find our solid ground when we have crossed shaky terrain. The cultivation of resilience is the most important embodied personal skill we can invest in.

In the erotic mapping process, resilience shows up as a bridge (see Figure 8.2) constructed of personal protective factors that allow us the choice to hinge back toward mastery when challenge presents itself instead of following a habitual thought and movement pattern into dysregulation and shadow. It is resilience that allows us to enter the *flow state* where our abilities are successfully meeting and overcoming the challenges of the environment. One of my workshop participants, Melissa Tilleman of Cambium Counseling, said that finding the flow state through resilience feels like finding the *hero dirt* on a mountain bike trail.

> *The beautiful viscosity of bound flow is like hero dirt when you're mountain biking. Hero dirt typically occurs when the soil has experienced rainfall or moisture in the last 24 hours. The dirt is neither muddy and slick nor dry and dusty. Instead, the dirt has the perfect tackiness to allow your mountain bike tires to hook up in such a dynamic way that you are able to be more playful and creative with the riding lines you choose while going down the trail. You can trust that your bike tires will hold their*

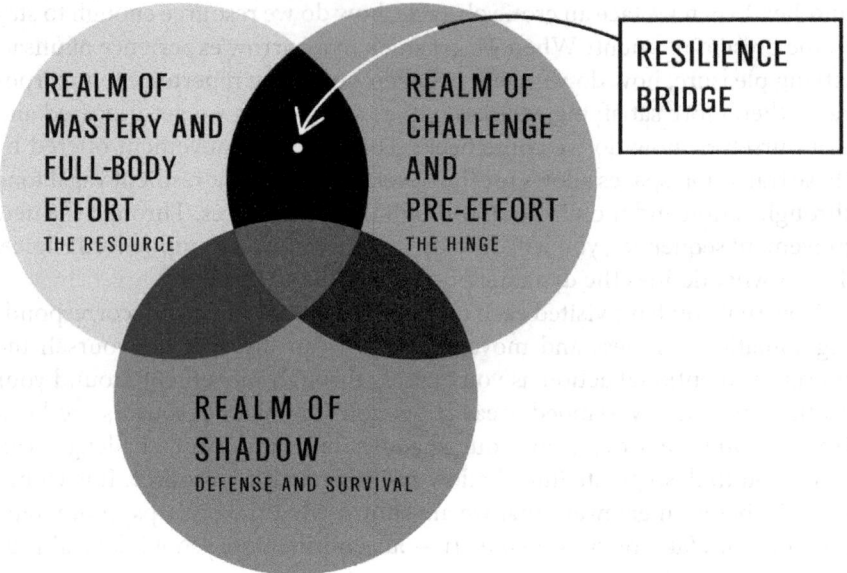

Figure 8.2   Resilience Bridge on the Erotic Map

> *line when you are leaning into a berm or going off a jump. It increases your sense of presence and oneness with your body, bike, the trail, and the surrounding terrain, which helps to put you in a state of playful and dynamic flow. It is the best!*

As an off-road bicyclist, Melissa is continually in search of the trail that provides that perfect Velcro-like traction, keeping her stable yet able to glide through corners and down hills. Resilience is the hero dirt.

Uncovering Your Resilience

Refer back to your movements in both the full-effort and challenge realms. Begin in the place of challenge and take time to embody the movement and breath you recorded. Now, transition into your full-effort or resource movement. Then return to your challenge movement. As you transition between the challenge to the resource movement, closely notice what your body is doing to get you there. What is the breath quality that helps you open and expand into full, congruent effort? Do you notice that a full out-breath and a shake-it-out quality must happen first? Try shaking, jumping, swaying, undulating, patting your whole body down with your hands . . . find what movement quality is satisfying. Is your chin lifted high or your mouth held tight, keeping you in the mind and away from

> *integration with your body? Soften your chin to your chest as your out-breath releases your jaw. We all have restorative movements that serve to regulate the nervous system via the soft tissues of the body. Just as the fawn that shakes off the freeze response after the mountain lion gives up the chase, your body knows what it needs to do to release the stress and bring you back into balance. Take your time and get to know the breath and movement qualities that work as a bridge from challenge back into resource.*
>
> *Once you have found satisfaction in your restorative movements, move your way into your mastery movement and embody it with full breath. Embody the mastery movement like you really mean it, starting small and gradually inviting the movement to increase, until warmth and ease spreads through your body.*
>
> *You have just created your resilient bridge sequence composed of three parts: challenge movement, bridging restorative movements, and mastery movement. Repeat this sequence multiple times to store it in your body memory.*

Dysregulation: Reactive Habitual Movement Patterns

Between the realm of challenge and the Pandora's box of shadow is an overlapping space (see Figure 8.3) that contains the dysregulated reactions that consume us in times of great stress and shame. When our challenge throws us out of our window of tolerance, we are overwhelmed and "hinge" into maladaptive coping strategies. These coping strategies are somatically imprinted as body armor—the protective gear written into our muscles and tissues in response to negative sexuality messages, personal trauma, transgenerational trauma, and the weight of the suppression of the best parts of us.

While these strategies may have, at one time, protected us from emotional or physical pain, these strategies no longer apply to our current life. Instead, they now hinder our relationship with ourselves and limit our ability to connect with intimate partners. It is not our fault that we have developed these reactions. Yet thankfully our body does have the tools to rewrite this automatic response, or at least to regulate ourselves out of this emotional and psychophysiological energy drain. It is important that we recognize when our experience of the challenge realm drops us into the shadow realm so that we can be awake to our reactivity and, therefore, hinge out of shadow back through the portal of resilience.

We must also make note of what current environments feel safe enough and supportive enough to hinge out of our coping strategies to begin with. Environments can help us feel safe and relaxed when we are stressed—they can also stress us out and prevent us from connecting with even our most

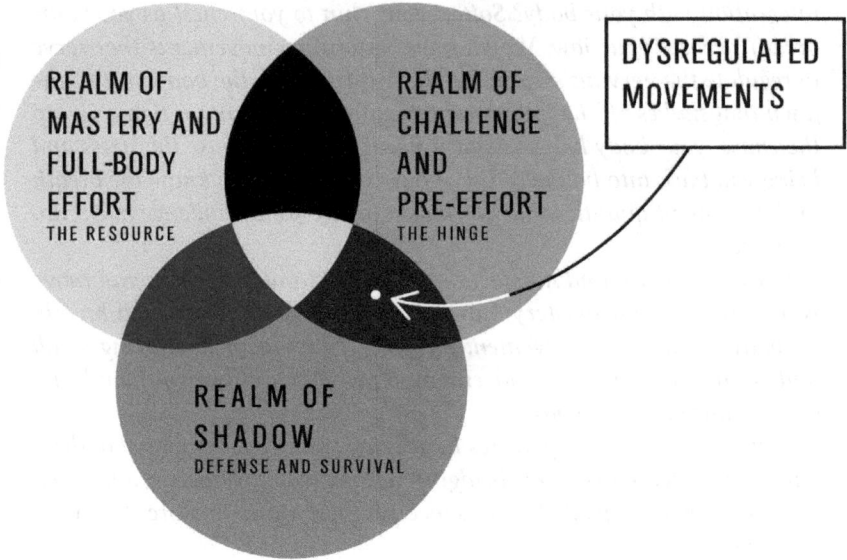

Figure 8.3   Dysregulated Movement Pattern of the Erotic Map

readily acceptable delights. Try enjoying Disneyland while fighting with a partner about your in-laws. No amount of cotton candy or smiling fairy-tale characters will make you genuinely happy here. Notice what elements of your environment allow you to hinge out of the shadow. Important elements that my clients have shared include relational elements like a partner who is on board with supporting without pressuring them to heal, being able to use their voice to state a boundary, or physical factors like being physically warm or not too hungry. The environment becomes a scaffolding so that the individual can have the best shot possible to put their skills of regulation to the task.

Identifying the Reactive Habitual Movement Pattern

Before you begin, return to your resource movement. Take your time to be filled up by this resilient movement and breath sequence. Also explore how you transitioned between the challenge movement back into the resource movement. We're about to drop into the next layer deeper and the work you have done to find resilience in the face of challenge is a blueprint. This practice is most effective when we titrate—visit the shadow realm for a few moments and then return to your resourcing movements. Over time, as you refine your ability to explore the shadowy underworld and find your way back out, you can increase the time spent exploring.

This practice is about touching into your shadow rather than plunging headfirst, so I encourage that you take this slow. If we blow past our boundaries, we will not be able to digest the wisdom and insight found here.

Let's begin.

Keeping your resource at the ready, allow yourself to visualize a time most recently when you experienced a strong feeling of guilt, shame, discomfort, anger, pain, or anxiety. Visualize the environment: who was there, what was happening, how you responded.

Take a breath. Invite your awareness to your quality of attention. Do your thoughts have a judgmental, critical, or "tunnel vision" quality to them? Take another intentional breath. Where in your body landscape do you feel tight or constricted muscles? Do you also notice any numbness or avoidance in any body locations? What movement qualities do you notice? Quick, furtive movements, a pulling in, a wanting to run out of the room, constriction in your throat or brow?

Invite another intentional breath and drop the visualization. Return to your resource or resilient movements—patting down your limbs or shoulders, shaking, stomping your feet, swaying. Find someone close and trusted to get a hug or describe your experience.

Eroticism Frozen in the Reach and Grasp

When we are stuck in the liminal space between shadow and resource (see Figure 8.4), we are in the realm of the hungry ghost. This hungry ghost has a belly the size of a mountain and a mouth the size of the eye of a needle—never able to take in enough to satisfy its cavernous longing. This erotic gateway, like an eddy in the river, contains the aspects of sexuality that are on autopilot or repeat in a looping gesture of unconscious reaching and grasping. Out of control sexual behavior specialist Douglas Braun-Harvey emphasizes that "all appetitive behaviors can spiral out of control—seeking satisfaction without responsibility, engaging in repetitive patterns that are harmful—bringing serious consequences and becoming less and less pleasurable as they become more and more automatic and excessive" (Braun-Harvey & Vigorito, 2015, pg. ix). This stagnant corner of the masterful, full-body effort realm of their erotic map contains a paint-by-numbers sexual sequence that gets us to orgasm, the same erotic film, the same vibrator we use, the same substance we use, or the parts of ourselves we unequivocally keep hidden.

While these things in and of themselves are not problematic, they become problematic when we reach for them without thinking or we most often use them in place of an intimate relationship and connection. Instead of accessing curiosity, present-moment attention, and life-giving creativity, we engage

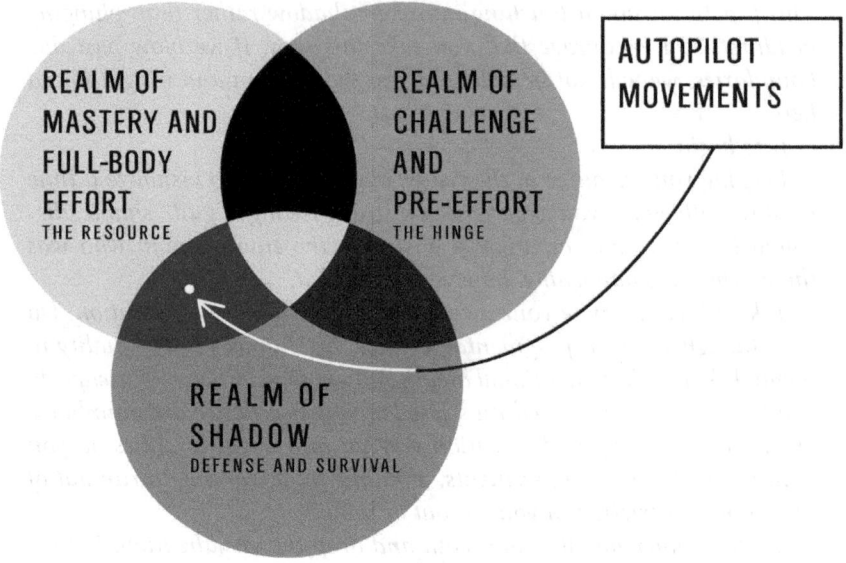

Figure 8.4 Autopilot Movement on the Erotic Map

in unsatisfying sexual behavior because it is *easy* or obvious and suppress any skepticism or dissatisfaction we may experience. Like entering a car wash, we go through the same steps of rolling up all the windows before driving our car onto the tracks as we are carried through the soaping, rinsing, and spot-free wash process. Through the efficient automation of modern invention, none of our muscles or attention is involved in this process. Just as neglecting body movement can atrophy our muscles, pleasure autopilot can atrophy eroticism. I want to note that this type of stagnancy is *different* than when someone has a need for safety and predictability due to past experiences of sexual trauma. The need for safety and moment-to-moment embodied consent is an alive and vital process. And this kind of erotic autopilot is unconscious and rigid.

When the approach to dealing with the challenge and shadow realms is to avoid or suppress difficulty, the realm of mastery can become a place where we get stuck in a Groundhog Day loop. As we repeat the activities that we enjoy and that give us pleasure with a narrow focus and bound-tension flow, we start to develop somatic rigidity and may develop obsessiveness, or what Braun-Harvey has termed *out of control sexual behavior* (OCSB). It's what "works" for us, though it is never fully satisfying and can damage valuable relationships, so we keep doing it instead of challenging ourselves to go deeper or to broaden our sexual repertoire. As we reach for what we want from a peripheral origin point (instead of reaching from a grounded place within us), the satisfaction we experience becomes diminished over time. We are reaching for more and more, yet are unable to truly breathe it in or rest into the pleasure.

Awakening the Automated Sexual Self

What are the activities that you find yourself participating in automatically? Automatic participation is reaching for something before taking the time to check in with yourself to sense what is truly wanted in the moment. Do you find that you automatically reach for the chocolate after a long day at work, even if it is not what your body is truly craving? Do you initiate sex with your partner the same way every time? Does sex follow a predictable pattern in most of your sexual encounters? Do you find yourself watching erotic videos or viewing erotic images (pornography) in the majority of your solo sex sessions? Is there a belief that you have about sex or your gender or sexual orientation that feels like a sweeping assumption or absolutist statement (men/women/committed couples do/ don't do X, Y, Z)? Select something that feels the most visceral to you.

As you visualize this activity or belief, notice what happens with your breath, your sensations, and your emotions. Notice where your center of gravity is. Do you feel off-balance, internally leaning too far this way or that? Where do you find your attention getting stuck? Do you find yourself spacing out, thinking about the grocery list or what you will do on your next day off? Let your in-breath call your attention back into your body. Exaggerate the small or large movements that you found yourself making during your visualization. As you repeat and clarify this movement, describe the sensory and movement qualities to yourself. Ask yourself if this feels familiar. Take a moment to write your experience in your journal.

Return again to your full-effort resource movement, softening your jaw and shoulders and inviting in a more full-body breath. Build the movement transition between the full-effort movement and the automated movement. Emphasize what movement qualities call your conscious awareness and sensory aliveness back to the forefront.

Spiraling Toward the Center: You Are All of This

The intersection of the full-effort, challenge, and shadow realms of the erotic map is where we find our core erotic self—a self that we can strive to embody more and more within the intimate realms where we feel safe enough to feel and express the deepest facets of our erotic aliveness. When the three realms of the erotic map are pressed together, the alchemical interaction is potent and compelling.

It is at this center where our *core erotic theme* resides (see Figure 8.5). Sex therapist and author Jack Morin defined the core erotic theme as the essence of your peak erotic experiences and fantasies. Morin identified this equation as Attraction + An Obstacle = *Core Erotic Theme* (1996). Attraction, the first part of the equation, is the free-flow rhythm of arousal energy. The obstacle creates bound-flow rhythm in the body. Taken together, the interplay between attraction and obstacles is the mechanism by which we integrate the unrealized potential of the erotic body. The more we learn and integrate, the more access we have to the vast terrain of the erotic.

When we engage our somatic skills at the border where arousal meets body armor—where the arousal of attraction meets the obstacle of the taboo or shadow—we experience our eroticism living in its most potent form. In other words, the erotic map shows us how Mastery + Challenge + Shadow = Core Erotic Theme. This is where our excitement peaks and our somatic mastery keeps us balanced, awake, and aware in order to study and savor the most compelling erotic experiences.

The potency of energy that makes up the core erotic self is that which connects us with the experience of others in the form of archetypal constructs. Archetypes are the enduring roles and personas that we humans all have an

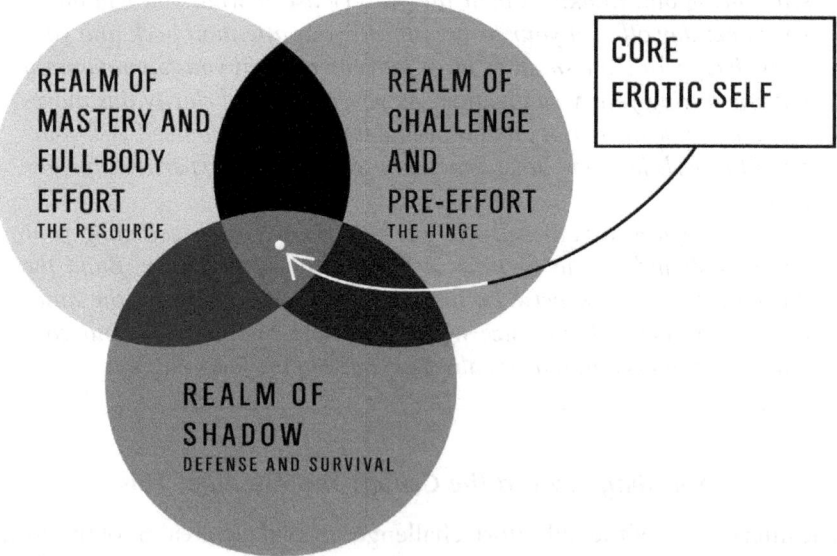

Figure 8.5 Core Erotic Self on the Erotic Map

experience of in our lives and relationships. The mother, the father, the lover, the youth, the martyr, the magician—these are all roles that we know intimately in our own way yet connect us all through a common identification of experience. When we arrive at our core erotic self, we arrive at our core archetypal aspects.

When earlier humans across the globe, from Greeks to Indigenous Americans, began identifying patterns in the stars, they quickly attributed these constellations to characters in their mythological stories. Of course they did—the human body is built for pattern recognition and from patterns emerge stories, meaning. We see ourselves in everything—anthropomorphizing stars, animals, and other natural features. We thrive on stories, symbolic and meaningful tales that give us a purpose, guidance, and reflection of our emotional struggles and triumphs. When we feel lost, stories give us a place-ness as we witness the journey of a protagonist. In *Women Who Run With the Wolves*, storyteller Clarissa Pinkola Estes (1996) reveals the importance of mythology to "sharpen our sight so that we can pick out and pick up the path left by the wildish nature. The instruction found in the story reassures us that the path has not run out, but still leads . . . deeper, and more deeply still, into their own knowing" (pg. 6). These are the archetypes with whom we can resonate—the personified subjects of story. After all, we do our most potent learning in relationship with other human beings or the natural world—whether in person or in the printed word.

Common archetypes that we all have some experience with are woven into our daily lives. We all have an experience of mother/father, child/adolescent, elder/crone, martyr/savior, for example. Stories of archetypes are contained within our movies, music, religious texts, and children's books. Parables, fairy tales, and mythology are teeming with age-old accounts of these patterns of tragedy, challenge, reclamation, and inspiration.

Archetypes are useful in working with the sexual self for three reasons. First, when we can see ourselves reflected in the world, we are no longer alone in our struggles. It can be a comforting feeling to know that we are not alone, that many others share our experience. Second, archetypes offer a clear picture of what is needed to move beyond challenges. When we are stuck in the moment and unable to see our way out of a problem, archetypal stories reveal a larger map and allow us to glimpse a reality beyond our struggles in the moment. Lastly, while stereotypes are spoken in a reductionistic and judgmental voice, archetypes are in fact expansive. They allow us to see our story on a grander scale. Not only are we not alone and have a map to refer to for guidance, we can find that our struggle is meaningful.

As I explore the erotic mapping process with my clients, core archetypes inevitably emerge and offer guidance to what is inhibiting or enhancing their erotic experience. Jungian sex therapist Chelsea Wakefield (Ogden, 2015) employs archetypes to assist in the journey of sexual individuation by exploring identities that are either Eros-enhancing or Eros-inhibiting. By identifying the archetypes standing in the foreground of the core erotic self, we are given a pathway to follow—somatically, emotionally, and psychologically.

As you explore your erotic map, what do you notice about the Eros-inhibiting aspects that have surfaced? Do you find yourself *mothering* or *fathering* your partner and therefore lacking sexual desire toward them? Or do you find that you recoil from deepening into an emotional sexual connection as the ever-adolescent more modern archetype of *Peter Pan*, who flies at the first hint of adulting? Do you sacrifice your needs and desires as a *martyr* in an attempt to maintain your relationship status quo? Perhaps you find sexual satisfaction through seeing your partner's pleasure in response to your successful *performer* skills yet have little to no connection to pleasure through receiving. These are the archetypes in their shadow aspects, the parts of self that are unconscious and therefore needing transformation to reveal your inhibited potential.

On the flip side, what do you notice about the Eros-enhancing aspects of your erotic map foreground (though they may have receded to the background)? Do you slink and smolder in your *siren* qualities as you call your lover to you, savor the groundedness in your muscles in your full-bodied *warrior* when you embrace your partner from a place of strength and *guardianship*, or feel wild abandon as you self-pleasure in your *virgin* solo sex practice ("virgin" in this context means self-to-self relationship versus self-to-other relationship)? These are some archetypes alive in their light aspects—the parts of self that are awake and embodied.

If you have trouble identifying Eros-enhancing archetypes, it is time to embark on your own journey to find an embodied archetype that feels intriguing and pleasurable to you. Explore your favorite movies from your youth, your favorite novels, or mythological characters. Comb through your divination cards and fairy tales. Through story, the archetypes who have wisdom for us will be revealed.

Once you find the archetype that is most interesting to you, take some time relating to this character. When I explored characters from adolescence with my client Ramona, she identified Belle from *Beauty and the Beast* as an archetype that attracted her from her earliest memories. Smart, strong, and with the ability to love what is fearful to others, Ramona felt a kinship with this heroine. Ramona felt others looked down their noses at her participation in polyamory, seen by her friends and family as an unwieldy *beast* that threatened the safety of their community. As I guided her to embody Belle, in posture, movement, and speech, Ramona connected with her long spine and fierce gaze. From this somatic foundation, she validated her draw to multiple partners as a growth-enhancing form of relationship.

The Dance of the Core Erotic Self

Now is the moment to combine the embodied movements from all three realms with their bridges as you loop this sequence into itself multiple times. Like the chorus of the song or primary guitar riff repeating itself to emphasize the underlying theme of the music, repeat this sequence so that the transitions become seamless. Mastery resource movement weaves into the challenge movement weaves into the shadow movement weaves into the mastery resource movement. Like the snake that eats its tail, the ouroboros, the end of the cycle feeds the beginning of the next cycle. Just as death feeds life, when we loop this movement sequence like an ouroboros, the shadow itself feeds our full-effort expression.

Notice what feels familiar to you when you string your movements together in a three-part sequence. What does this feeling and progression of movements remind you of? A character from your favorite movie or book? A person from your life? Make a note of their qualities before you continue to the next section.

Applying Your Erotic Map to Your Life

You now have both a visual and a somatic map to explore, to learn from, and to reorient you when you become lost or stuck. Begin by putting your movement sequence into action as a morning movement meditation, preparing yourself for whatever may happen during the day. You could also explore your movement sequence with a trusted friend, group, or counselor to invite the gems to shimmy to the surface with the support of a witness. Make sure that this is someone who can hold a compassionate, nonjudgmental space while reflecting your strengths to you. When you engage in a creative activity or an erotic encounter, let your breath and total-body connectivity of your mastery movement send your enjoyment to new heights. And when you get stuck in a shadowy place, intentionally revisit your resilient movements to bridge you into a more grounded exploration of your challenge. When you are ready, you can invite a partner to overlap their erotic map with yours.

9

THE RELATIONSHIP CONSTELLATION

Interweaving Erotic Maps

When we think of sex, we most often think of it as a partner dance—a sexy, amorous play space that includes you and one or more others. While solo sex is a wonderous and valid form of sex, sharing in mutual pleasure gets the most airtime for good reason: we are fundamentally social beings and the exchange of sexual energy with others can fuel our vitality and our sense of feeling *complete*. We feel vibrant, we feel loved, and we feel whole.

But the meeting of two sexualities can also be marked by stress, anxiety, and misunderstanding. Do you find that you spend time making assumptions about each other rather than being in the present moment together? Instead of curiosity, do you find that you idealize, mistrust, or shut out the vast terrain of your partner's eroticism? Shortcutting your beliefs about your partner's sexuality impedes the ability to deepen with that partner. This, in turn, impedes learning and depth experience in the relationship.

When practiced with a committed or consensual play partner, whole-body sexuality is a powerful opportunity to strengthen the experience of loving and being loved, to give and receive pleasure, and to deepen your bond with yourself while deepening the bonds of a relationship. This is sex and intimacy as a contemplative practice—an agreement to be in the present moment, to be responsible for one's own reactions and thoughts, and to refine the ability to connect with our direct experience as we resonate with the experience of another.

In Chapter 8, we explored your individual erotic map, the individualized constellation of your sexual mastery, challenges, and shadows. By overlapping your erotic map with the map of a partner, relationship patterns begin to emerge, revealing how you inspire and challenge each other as well as what personal shadows become activated by your dynamic together. Practicing

DOI: 10.4324/9780429297236-10

the vital components that comprise sexual embodiment together, while collectively exploring your erotic maps, creates a wonderful environment for healing and inspirational intimacy.

Four Pillars of Embodied Intimacy: Preparing to Combine Erotic Maps

First, let us explore how to cultivate an optimal environment around your relationship before laying out the process for combining erotic maps. This optimal environment includes practicing four pillars of embodied intimacy and striving for mutual total-body connectivity within your partnership. This is not about becoming masterful *before* entering an intimate relationship. If we waited until we totally knew ourselves and felt totally embodied, we would be waiting for a very long time. Instead, these components are ways of being that we can practice daily, to the best of our ability, for the rest of our lives. Relationship is an ongoing opportunity to study ourselves and our experiences, to better ourselves, and to carry forward the bright gems from our families of origin while evolving beyond the shadows of our lineage.

While you combine your erotic maps, it is helpful to practice some skill-building with your partner to fortify your foundation. We all have the responsibility to contribute to our relationships to the best of our ability. We can't just *wait for a partner to change*. Every relationship is a dynamic—a co-creation between people that is specific to you and your partner(s). When you strive for good relationship skills, you have the power to shift a dynamic. When you and your intimate other agree to practice these skills, something truly wonderful and transformative takes place. Mutual trust and appreciation for each other's efforts increases as relationship satisfaction grows. While the transition to better relationship habits can be challenging, it is worth it.

The four pillars of embodied intimacy include self-awareness, communication and expressiveness, sexual intelligence, and a balance between safety and novelty.

Pillar One: Self-Awareness With a Partner

Know Thyself. This ancient Greek aphorism inscribed on the Temple of Apollo in Delphi encourages timeless guidance on being human. The more willing you are to cultivate awareness of yourself in important moments, the more you can positively impact your relationships without leaving yourself behind. One of the temptations here is to believe that to *know thyself* means that you stand by unchanging traits and behaviors. While there are aspects of our personality that endure through the years, we have an underlying *organicity*, an orientation toward growth and change (Kurtz, 1990). In addition to the information that you have gathered from your personal erotic map, an important part of knowing yourself is to recognize how you engage with the natural process of change. As you cultivate a relationship to change—an awareness and appreciation for growth, cycles, and rhythms—you learn to approach new or challenging relationship dynamics with a resilience that heralds more positive outcomes.

The central focus of this pillar is to combine the information that you know about yourself and your sexuality with an ability to regulate your emotional body enough to communicate with your partner effectively. The self-directed practices that strengthen this first pillar include whole-body awareness (from sensation to quality of thoughts), erotic bodyfulness practice (as discussed in Chapter 4), awareness and validation of your own emotions and desires, identifying your defensive and protective reactions, and practicing the skills to modulate yourself within your window of tolerance through self-regulation of your nervous system and emotions. The window of tolerance is the range of nervous system activation that allows for best-effort participation in relationship—not enough activation leaves you shut down or depressed, while too much activation releases a tidal wave of ungrounded high intensity. While dropping out of the window of tolerance is a normal human experience, we can refine the ability to shift back into our window of tolerance. Maybe we get so mad that we can't think, and then we calm ourselves down. Or maybe we get so sad that we don't want to get out of bed, and then we cheer ourselves up. How each of us modulates, how long it takes, and how it impacts our relationships varies greatly between us, so learning what works for you is the key. This key gives you the empowered ability to contribute more of your beautiful, tender, inspiring self to a relationship.

Knowing yourself also includes learning about how your sociocultural identity impacts the way you relate with a partner. Understanding that you and your partner exist in different bodies, are from different families, and may be from a different intersection of sociocultural factors and therefore have had different experiences is vital to seeing your role in relationship on a deeper, more systemic level. This includes awareness of the role you play in power and gender dynamics, your beliefs about personal and relationship priorities, and your expression of emotions and desires, among other aspects.

Pillar number one questions to ask yourself are: What do you know about your own erotic map? What turns you on, turns you off, calms you down, or aggravates you? What kind of relationship did your parents, stepparents, grandparents, etc. model for you? What is your history of touch? What brings out the best in you or the worst in you? How do you respond to your partner when they are at their best and how do you respond to them when they are at their worst? How do you embody your gender in your relationship? What are the relationship values you have absorbed from your location in society (class, age, ability, race, ethnicity, state/country/region, religion, etc.)?

Pillar Two: Expressiveness With a Partner

Interact with a partner as you embody self-awareness (pillar one) and you have arrived at pillar number two. This is where you learn about how you understand, communicate, and express with intimate others. Making room for your experience and the experience of a partner is an art—a complex dance of competing and resonating bodies full of needs, values, and personal styles. Regardless of personal differences, you can co-create an open, curious, and trusting space to share your sexuality.

First, learning how to shift from a defensive state (fighting or avoiding challenge) into a receptive state (engaging and leaning into challenge) fuels a more easeful connection with a partner. This shift is effective when you have a good sense of the workings of your own nervous system, an awareness that you both have different bodies and experiences, and a toolbox of effective communication skills. Receptiveness and defensiveness have corresponding body states that alert you to which state you are in. Often, what looks defensive to one partner is actually an attempt at protecting a vulnerable part of themselves. Tune your awareness to what your body is trying to do for you when in a protective or defensive posture and share with your partner what is being protected. Notice how the *somatic markers* (Damasio, 1994) of your somatic landscape, like little tags marking sensory and movement stuck points, indicate defensiveness and receptiveness.

Generally, defensiveness is experienced as tightness in the jaw, chest, or abdomen, a closed body posture, constricted facial muscles, and a narrowing of the body *away* from a partner. This can be accompanied by a general lack of body awareness or awareness of self. Meanwhile, receptiveness is experienced as softness or openness in the chest and abdomen, an open body posture, soft or wide facial expressions, and a leaning *toward* a partner.

Professor of psychology Barbara Fredrickson (2013) refers to this receptive synchrony as *positivity resonance*, a shared moment of love, mirroring of movement, and a deep sense of caring for each other. Positivity resonance builds on itself and can sustain a relationship over time. On your own, practice shifting your body between defensive and receptive postures so that you know what you need to be able to turn back toward a partner: a strong out-breath, a wide stretch, and a shaking of the body like a rag doll followed by a deep and expansive in-breath are some of the ways to transition into receptivity.

Defensive states are a normal and important experience, directing you to listen to the important feelings and body memories that want to be explored.

Shifting into receptivity does not mean that you relinquish the importance of your own feelings; it just means you will be in a better mind-body state to communicate to them and be heard.

In addition to somatically shifting your emotional state, *how and what* you communicate can determine whether you get the best response from a partner. In *Emotional Intelligence in Couples Therapy* (2005), couples therapist Brent Atkinson describes the main components of effective communication skills to practice with a partner. These are the components: avoid erroneous fault-finding (don't jump to conclusions); find the "understandable part" (the part of your partner's experience that makes sense to you); identify your partner's underlying needs, values, and worries; offer assurance that you're doing your best to hear your partner with an open mind; give and ask for equal regard (both of your feelings are just as important and valid); and stand up for yourself without making a "big deal" about it. These communication skills support you and your partner to shift brain states from a *defensive* mode back into a *receptive* mode. Atkinson emphasizes that "the internal states that propel attack-defend escalations are not compatible with the habits that predict relationship success" (pg. 125). Shifting into a receptive brain state allows you to be open to your partner so that you can lean in, pick up on more nuance, and see them just as they are.

The second aspect of pillar two is to question your automatic thoughts about your partner's beliefs and behaviors and, instead, meet them with interest. Taking the time to halt your assumptions about your partner while bringing your curiosity to their actual, lived experience reaps huge rewards—they will be more open to you and you will get to learn what is really going on for them. My client Isabelle brightened when I described this to her and her husband, Lucas. "It's like peeking at the real person behind the curtain! Even though we've been together for so long, we still fixate on the curtain instead of asking to see what's really in each other's hearts." For example, if a partner seems nervous while sharing a desire, this might automatically appear to you as an indicator of them being untrustworthy. But what if it were actually excitement mixed with shame, embarrassment, or uncertainty? Or, if a partner is not sharing much detail and is in a closed body posture, you may think that they are withholding something. But what if, in reality, they are feeling fear because their sharing of a sexual interest in a prior relationship was met with anger? Share with each other your heart behind the curtain; where there is a rupture, there can be a repair. Each exchange about things like desires is an opportunity to meet each other with openness and to be rewarded with genuine connection.

Lastly, co-create an atmosphere that is safe enough to express movement and emotion with each other. It will be crucial for both of you to pay attention to what is expressed through the body: it is a wealth of important information and is thus a valuable resource. We are much less likely to share ourselves when we are afraid that we will be judged or labeled. Placing value on genuine expression, even when it is challenging or uncomfortable, gets us to the truth and back into connection much quicker than talking circles around each other. Explore together the movement patterns that hint at your broader relationship themes.

Questions to ask yourself here at pillar two are: What do you pay attention to about your partner's behaviors, priorities, and values? What do you value in relationship (or not)? Does your partner share these values (or not) and do they have a similar or different way of demonstrating them? What types of things do you verbalize to your partner or withhold? What emotions do you allow yourself to express and which ones do you withhold? What emotions or emotional range do you value or denounce in your partner? How much and what kind of touch do you enjoy with your partner and do they share this touch preference? Note that the answer to these questions is influenced by family dynamics, cultural stereotypes, and biases about gender roles, family roles, etc., as well as prior intimate relationship experiences.

Pillar Three: Embodied Sexual Wisdom With a Partner

Pillar number three highlights the aspect of yourself that is at the core of this book: embodied sexuality. Your sexuality can be a personal strength in relationship—one that supports mutual satisfaction and a deeper bond. Just like anything else, wisdom related to your sexuality requires an openness to learning and time to practice. This third pillar encourages understanding one's own erotic map, acquiring accurate information about arousal anatomy and studying your own body, practicing responsibility over the activation and direction of your sexual arousal, and learning what you need in order to access a space of curiosity and playfulness when exchanging desires with a partner.

First, begin by exploring yourself *for yourself*. When we only explore our desire and sexual response in relationship to partner sex, we only learn about ourselves as a member of a dynamic; in this dynamic, the comingling of desires and expectations naturally take center stage. Make sure you set aside solo time to fantasize, self-pleasure, and engage in other sexual or nonsexual pleasurable activities. Notice how your body responds to arousing stimulation without needing to address the desires of a partner. Approach this solo learning time like a fascinated scientist—you are not trying to make anything specific happen. Instead, you are approaching your body with wonder and genuine interest. Take time to appreciate and celebrate your body. As you learn about yourself, you will have self-knowledge and sexual self-confidence to benefit your more-than-one sexual play.

Then, you can carry your awareness, questions, and new learning into partner sex and notice what happens when your body erotically meets with another. For example, how is your orgasm, your voice quality, your body movement different or similar when you are with a partner versus with yourself? What does this tell you about your erotic map—your areas of mastery, challenge, and shadow? Sex with yourself and sex with another becomes a co-informing, co-creating symphony.

Second, practice speaking about your knowledge of your sexual self with a trusted partner. This allows you to be more comfortable with verbalizing, and therefore validating, your experiences. Increasing verbal ease in sharing information about yourself with a partner, as well as asking about their experience, paves the road to more ease and freedom in your sexual relationship. Challenges are more easily addressed, and pleasure is more freely enjoyed, when we co-create a safe space to dialogue.

Lastly, practicing embodied touch is an important component of accessing sexual wisdom with a partner. Invite and offer contact of each other's bodies while training your awareness like a dowsing rod toward pleasure. See Chapter 7 for a discussion on embodied touch.

Pillar Four: Balance Between Safety and Novelty With a Partner

As previously stated from the work of neuroscientist Stephen Porges, we need a certain measure of safety to be in proximity for touch, bonding, and ultimately for good sex. Physical safety is not enough—we must also have enough emotional safety to feel curious, to be conscious, to be embodied, and to be turned on by erotic touch.

Yet, too much safety and security leads to erotic disaster. Relationship therapist Ester Perel draws attention to the paradox of love and desire. Love wants closeness, familiarity, and safety, while desire wants novelty, risk, and spontaneity. Many of my clients recall a time, often in the beginning of their relationship, where sex was easier and more effortless. This period of time most often includes a relationship structure that had a built-in balance between individual time and together time. For example, they didn't live together so they only saw each other on the weekends or for a lunch date with a "quickie" in the car. Once people live together, combining lives and responsibilities, they begin to feel more like family and less like an exciting, new adventure. As love deepens, novelty recedes. Too often, we drop into habits that do not support intimacy, though they do facilitate the efficiency of day-to-day life. *You take the kids to the park and I'll get the groceries. You plan the vacation and I'll give you the credit card. You watch your TV show downstairs while I read in the bedroom.* Sometimes working efficiently as a team can lead to functioning almost completely independently of each other. While splitting duties and activities is helpful to the relationship and supports a continued sense of self, it can also puncture a couple's sense of connection.

While some relationships become parallel lives, I see other relationships take a path of entanglement where people have pushed their own needs and desires to the side because they think this will increase the safety and security of their partnership. You finally get that date night and spend the evening talking about the mortgage, the kids, or your job. You no longer participate in cherished hobbies, the kind that activate your passionate self, and instead sit on the couch with your partner as they watch their favorite show. Instead of increasing security, devaluing your passions dampens your life spark and builds resentment over time.

It may feel risky, but it is important to emphasize *intimacy over efficiency* while working on the foundation of a relationship. Instead of taking the efficient shortcut, what would increase your sense of aliveness within yourself and with a partner? Slowing down for intimacy, as clunky as it may feel in the beginning, opens real relationship depth and a more satisfying ebb and flow of diverging and converging erotic paths. This is a practice of incorporating risk in a way that feeds eroticism.

Playing with risk does not mean participating in activities that feel scary, the kind that give you a knot in your stomach and trigger the protective mechanisms of the body. The kind of risk that can benefit a relationship activates a mixture of excitement and nervousness or awkwardness, the sort of things found in the *challenge* area of your erotic map. It's more about introducing some novelty and adventure to your relationship—opportunities for your body-mind to access that optimal learning environment where your habitual movement patterns are challenged to adapt to a new situation or environment. Novelty can be a whole spectrum of things, like engaging in familiar sexual activity while including a bit of something new, taking a partner on a date to a new place, sharing sexual fantasies, or adventuring through sensation play (like alternating candle wax and ice cubes down your lover's back, change of intimate setting, role-play, etc.). With the other three pillars as support, you and your partner can find your way to grounded and connected intimacy through some edge-walking.

Another way to create the conditions for novelty is to invest in yourself through personal development, hobbies, passions, and time with the people and landscapes that bring out the best in you. This ensures that you are feeding the core of who you are and bringing revitalized energy back into your relationship.

Remember that novelty must be balanced with familiarity and connection, so make sure to prioritize meaningful time with your partner. It is the rhythm of *activation into rest* and *distance into closeness*—the in-breath and the out-breath—that tones and strengthens the connection between your nervous systems and hearts.

Combining Erotic Maps

With the four pillars of embodied intimacy as a foundation, we can begin to explore your personal erotic maps together to reveal your relationship strengths, challenges, and shadow dynamic. Reviewing the side-by-side erotic

map framework helps to identify the deeper themes that energize your relationship as well as the aspects that activate conflict. Because two people create a
system, combined erotic mapping is also an opportunity to consciously evaluate the larger sociocultural themes that you embody in your dynamic while
you improve your direct relationship. The discovery of those entrenched
familial or cultural relationship patterns lets you take control of the hidden
forces that have been influencing your behavior. As you engage in the process in the following sections, share with your partner what feels safe enough
to offer yet also pushes your edges. You do not need to begin by sharing
everything—instead, share what is within your window of tolerance and then
challenge yourself to share something edgy.

Share your mastery: After you and a partner complete your erotic maps
under the guidance of Chapter 8, set your maps in front of you as you sit
beside each other (see Figure 9.1). Begin by sharing your areas of mastery—
the places and activities where you feel grounded in your sexuality as well as
the associated sensations and movement. Invite your partner to mirror the
mastery movement that you clarified in your erotic map by trying on the
breath and gestures that you embody. Then invite your partner to share their
mastery areas, sensations, and movements and reflect their movement back
to them. Remember that you are not *mimicking* each other's movement; you

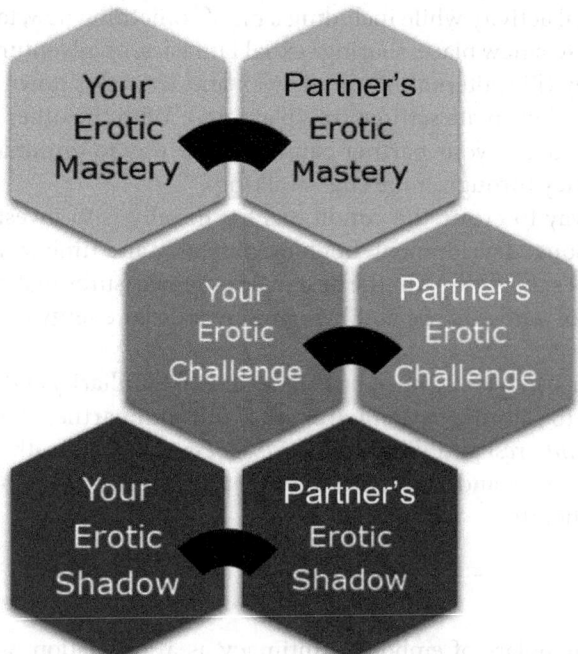

Figure 9.1 Combining Erotic Maps With a Partner

are trying on each other's expression to see how it feels in your own body and to join with your partner in the spirit of attunement. Sharing mastery movements doesn't have to be a stoic or serious exchange! This is a good place to invite play and laughter as you explore your movements long enough to refine pre-effort mirroring into full effort attunement.

Once you have both shared, practice connecting your movements and breath together, transitioning between both of your mastery movements to create a kind of call-and-response dance together. Perhaps your partner offered a jumpy, bubbly mastery movement while your movement was more grounded and fluid. As you practice transitioning between these two different movement profiles, what sort of breath and full-body gesture helps you soften from the bubbly jumping rhythm to drop into the fluid swaying rhythm? And what breath quality and movement gesture helps you lift up from the grounded fluidness into the more vertically oriented bubbly expression? Take your time exploring the transition.

You may notice that your partner's mastery movement feels attractive or exciting to you. You may also find that your partner's mastery movement feels uncomfortable to you. Both are normal here! If you find a sense of discomfort at this stage, you may find that your partner may have mastered something that is still living in your challenge or shadow areas. At this point, identify something that you know you enjoy together and share your sensations and gestures to find your combined mastery movement. This is your home base movement, the place where both of you feel comfortable and connected.

Before moving on, share what you notice here. Staying with description (nonjudgmental, observable, sensory language), share with each other how the experience impacted your somatic and emotional landscape. Tell your partner what you felt in your body—your sensation, emotion, and movement experience—while exploring your combined mastery movement. Close with specific and descriptive appreciations of each other.

Share your challenge: Your area of challenge contains the activities or aspects of your sexual self where you experience complex pleasure—a blend of interest or attraction combined with anxiousness or frustration. Share with your partner what you currently find challenging in your sexuality and the corresponding sensations, emotions, and movements that go with that frustration. As you and your partner embody your challenge aspects, you may recognize this from an area of your relationship. You most likely have seen your partner exhibit their challenge movements when they are stressed, when sex doesn't go so well, or at the tipping point of an argument. This is your opportunity to learn what is behind this response (remember that person behind the curtain?) so that you can better understand your partner and shift from a defensive to receptive response.

Ask each other about the movement bridge (the resilient breath and movement) that facilitates the shift from challenge to mastery so that you can witness each other transform from awkward or disorganized into a clearer expression. Notice here how your sense of mastery can support your partner's challenge or vice versa. I usually discourage my partnered clients from mirroring the challenge movements and instead simply say "thank you for sharing your challenge with me." Because the challenge area often contains a very personal frustration or an anxiety, I find that relationships are better served by one partner simply offering to witness to the other while offering nonjudgment and an open heart to the best of their ability. Practicing being seen in vulnerability sharpens your resilience and increases a sense of safety to tackle challenges together. Remember that we are more likely to take risks together if we feel safe. Close this section by sharing specific appreciations with each other.

Share your shadow: Before sharing the shadow area of your erotic maps, revisit your mastery movements together, linking up breath and movement to remember your resilience, then take turns sharing your shadow area and its corresponding sensations, emotions, and movements. You may recognize your partner's shadow movements from the times when they are in their darkest moments or when you were in a big conflict. It is possible that the expressions of mastery or challenge in one of you activates the shadow in the other. Support each other to shift back into the mastery movements that help you feel your resilience and offer appreciation to each other. This is the moment of sharing that holds the greatest vulnerability and therefore requires the slowest pace as well as the most emphatic reflections of love and support. Encourage each other to just dip a toe in here, to titrate, and then return to a grounding breath and mastery movement together.

Combine what you have learned: Now discuss together what you learned as you followed this process to co-create a *relationship erotic map*. What did you enjoy? What surprised you? What was the hardest part? At each step in the process, you learned what lights you both up, what presents obstacles to your sexual fulfillment as partners, and what induces desire discrepancies. You now get to place this information within a framework that helps you access awareness of your relationship dynamic and provides the somatic pathway to lead you out of dissonance into resonance.

In your area of *mastery*, write down the places and activities where you easily access your sexuality *together*. Make a note of the movements and postures that you each embody and express when you engage with each other in easeful pleasure. Do you find that your whole-body expression shows up when you play tennis together, engage in sexual play on vacation, or when you flirt over text before coming home? Securing the things that work well for both of you can be the touchstones you return to when the challenges and shadows of your relationship create too much uncertainty.

In your area of *challenge*, include the ways you interact where you feel interest or desire along with some sort of discomfort. Describe each of your movements and breath quality in detail. A challenge could be that you have a harder time getting into a sexy mood because you have toddlers or jobs that occupy most of your energy. Perhaps a partner's sexual interests cause you to feel uneasy or inadequate, or perhaps an injury or illness is impeding the expression of your sexuality in the way you want.

In the *resilience* space between challenge and mastery, list the things that help you emotionally and physiologically co-regulate so that you both know how to return to connection in the midst of challenging interactions. Your resilience dance could consist of immediate loving touch or it could consist of first regulating yourselves in your own way followed by loving touch or words with each other. Be as descriptive as possible in the movements, rhythms, and qualities of touch and breath that help you access resilience together.

In the area of overlap between challenge and shadow, write the things that hinge you deeper into conflict and make resilience more difficult. This is the ineffective coping mechanism dynamic that takes resolution farther out of reach. Remember, this is not about placing fault but about identifying what happens so that each of you can take a part of the responsibility and have the power to prevent dropping into shadow territory.

In your area of *shadow*, write down the realizations that you had about how your individual shadow appears in the relationship, how you activate each other's shadow, and how you may help each other out of the dark places. You may find that one of your shadows is counterbalanced by the other's mastery, allowing you to meet in the area of challenge for healing. For example, one of you may have learned that your self-worth relies on what you give others, therefore draining your energy and muting your own sexual expression. Meanwhile, your partner may find mastery in both giving and receiving pleasure and insist that you are valuable just as you are, not just when you are masterfully giving them pleasure. This allows you to feel safe enough to practice receiving pleasurable touch from your partner, though it may still feel edgy and awkward—because of this relationship dynamic, your shadow heals just enough to shift it into a manageable challenge.

It is possible that discomfort can arise when sharing personal erotic maps and that is an important part of the process. Emotional and physiological activation is like an alarm being raised to alert you to where good relationship work can be focused. However, by discovering your area of relationship mastery, you can leverage somatic co-creative resilience to bridge out of dissonance more quickly than you ever have before instead of getting stuck in the same old conflict again and again.

My clients Cary and Kennedy came in for solo sessions to map out their individual erotic constellations and then returned for a couple session to combine their maps and get a clearer picture of the source of their desire difference. Cary, a white, 36-year-old high-school teacher from Denver, found that he felt anxious about initiating intimacy. Meanwhile, Kennedy, a white, 40-year-old psychotherapist originally from Quebec, was struggling with feeling the desire for sex at all. In their combined mastery area, they learned that they both felt excited and sensual when they cooked on the weekends, with the music turned up loud and no work responsibilities to tend to. They got to laugh and dance together while enjoying delicious smells and sensual movements. I invited them to practice erotic bodyfulness to refine the breath and movement of their combined mastery movement. They breathed deeply as they pressed their hands together while swaying their hips. "Take a snapshot of this moment," I offered, "so we can come back to it."

Then we explored their challenge area: Cary's challenge appeared when he felt attracted to Kennedy and wanted to initiate sex. Warmth and tingling would rise in his stomach, but as soon as he moved to engage sexually, Cary felt his whole body constrict as he saw Kennedy lean away from his touch. Kennedy reported a strong stomach-constricting freeze response to Cary's reach. In her challenge area, she described seeing "that hunger" in Cary's eyes as he moved quickly to "grab" at an area of Kennedy's body.

As we explore the somatic relationship between their bodies in this moment by slowing down the typical interaction—Cary accessing attraction for Kennedy and then moving to touch her as Kennedy leaned her body away— we discover something very important that they'd never realized before. In the first few moments of Kennedy seeing Cary's attraction for her, Kennedy noticed she felt *excited*, but this quickly shifted into anxiety when Cary sped up with grabbing gestures. I pointed to Kennedy's shadow area: her first sexual experience with a boy who "rushed" her in a bathroom during class at their junior high. She had a crush on him and so she did not want to say "no" to his advances. At first, she was excited by his attention, but this quickly turned into a freeze response as he pushed her into a stall to continue his rapid advances. Kennedy felt assaulted and her crush on the boy turned into outright anxiety. As Kennedy fought back tears recalling this moment, sharp in-breaths and chin lifting high away from her body, I encouraged Cary to stand with his palms facing out. Kennedy understood immediately and stepped in to press her hands against Cary's as Cary began to gently sway. Kennedy's chin lowered toward her chest as her out-breath softened her shoulders with a long sigh. Before long, they pressed into each other, swaying together in a close embrace.

By moving toward their resilience movement, both were able to regulate, access a reparative experience, and return to connection. Cary also learned to slow his approach to his partner, giving Kennedy the time to enjoy her excitement and meet Cary in the middle for intimacy. While Cary was still the higher-desire partner, Kennedy now had more space to feel his desire and even be the one to initiate sometimes.

While this example contains a male-female heterosexual couple, I have seen a similar dynamic play out in a myriad of different couples with different gender dynamics and relationship structures.

Erotic Mapping for Non-monogamy and Polyamory

If you are non-monogamous, you may want to incorporate portions of the erotic map of multiple partners and how this impacts you and your other relationships. As you review the combined erotic map with a primary partner, include your combined mapping of another romantic or play partner. Multiple relationships are not separate from each other; the ripples of impact overlap and can highlight important elements to explore further—elements that might have previously been overlooked. You may find that a personal sexual mastery, while too challenging or uninteresting to one partner, is in the mastery area of another partner and so allows you to refine and deepen your experience of yourself with them. This abundance of energy fills you up so that you have more patience and excitement to support another partner in their challenge or shadow area. You may also find that a personal shadow is pressing you to seek out connection with another partner when things get challenging with a primary partner, thereby preventing conflict resolution and the integration of your shadow elements.

Embodied Sexuality for One Hot Minute

You may not be in a committed relationship, or you may be in a partnered non-monogamous relationship and you have agreed to engage in sexual connection outside of your primary relationship. Regardless, each sexual experience is a relationship, even when it is a temporary connection. While you may not be interested in diving deep into the nuances of your connection with this person, some fundamental principles of sexually relating to yourself and to another can still support a satisfying experience: ownership of your arousal, negotiating consent and desired activities, and respect of yourself and your sexual partners. According to Dossie Easton, author of *The Ethical Slut*:

> *A lot of people describe having sex with only one person as "being faithful." It seems to me that faithfulness has very little to do with who you have sex with. Faithfulness is about honoring your commitments and respecting your friends and lovers, about caring for their well-being as well as your own.*
>
> (Easton & Hardy, 2017, pg 63)

Have your erotic map in mind as you engage in sex with a new partner and fold it into your sexy flirtation and into a check-in about your sexual health. Here are some examples of how you can do this:

- Masterful: "What excites you the most about sex?" "Here's what excites me. . . ."
- Challenge: "Here's what I'm exploring about my sexuality right now. . . ." "What new things are you exploring with sex right now? Do you want to explore that with me?"
- Shadow: "What are you not into/what's your boundary right now?" "Here's what I don't feel comfortable exploring right now."
- Follow this up with what really excites you about them.

Desire Difference: When Erotic Maps Clash

At some point, everyone will experience desire difference with a partner. It is such a common dynamic. It can show up as a different preference in sexual frequency, preferred sexual activities, time of day for intimacy, or whether to open to other romantic or sexual partners. It can be disheartening when your erotic maps seem to conflict and contradict each other. However, a difference in desire does not have to signal the end of a relationship. By acknowledging the difference, taking the time to understand each other's desires, expanding the palette of how sex is defined, and exploring power dynamics, a discrepancy can be an opportunity for growth and deeper bonding. This section explores how to deal with a discrepancy that is beginning to dismantle your sense of connection.

Acknowledge the difference: Desire difference is normal and does not have to be a problem—it is an opportunity. I hear people question whether a desire difference means that they are not meant for each other or that they have grown apart. Actually, discrepancy is an indication that a couple has become stagnant in their relationship, that they are ready for the next level of relational or personal growth, or that they have misunderstood what one partner is requesting. It can also be an indication of contention in their underlying emotional attachment. By acknowledging that desire discrepancy is normal, the partners can set aside the existential questions to begin the problem-solving process as a team.

Take the time to understand: When desire difference shows up, partners often jump to conclusions, minimizing the sexual complexity of themselves and their partner. Friction from the mismatch builds, and partners end up venting absolutes and vague statements at each other: "I could have sex any-time!" or "I just want to be heard!" or "I just want sex to be passionate, or nat-ural, or [fill in the blank]!" The more I help people explore such statements, the more complexity we find, easing the urgency and paving the road to more accurate and feasible requests. By listening to your partner with curiosity and interest, you may find out that their desires are not as incongruous as you think, or you may realize that you misunderstood what they actually desire. This is not necessarily anyone's fault—you are in different bodies and have had different experiences and, therefore, interpret and express (or withhold) things differently. Each of you has a different somatic experience and mental image that activates when you talk about "sex" or "attraction" or "passion."

Additionally, you may find that you have oversimplified or misrepresented your own desires. Look to the challenge area of your erotic map to find the desires that you may be expressing in an incongruent or "mixed message" sort of way because it is a desire that you find interesting but which also creates a sense of nervousness or anxiousness in you. This can be confusing to a partner; help them understand your magnificent complexity.

Expand the definition of sex: Sex has been redefined throughout this book to include more than just intercourse, more than just oral sex, and far beyond what happens in the bedroom. Viewing sex as a multifaceted experience is one of the quickest ways to explore a desire discrepancy. When a whole palette of sexual and sensual activities is presented, sex becomes so much more than a series of positions or a frequency quota. Draw a circle on a piece of paper and write all the pleasure-focused activities that you and a partner enjoy. My colleague Jenni Skyler uses the metaphor of a cheesecake where each slice is a different flavor—all are equally delicious, yet they are qualitatively different. Include a range of sensual and sexual things: an appreciative gesture, kissing, flirtatious texting, erotic massage, penetrative sex, etc. If you do one of these things every day, your intimacy is successful. By shifting your perspective to include many presentations of sex, you will find that you have much more in common erotically with a partner than you think.

Power dynamics: Every relationship has a power dynamic. This dynamic includes the ways in which we get what we want and need by navigating the power-up and power-down position with an intimate other. This power dynamic is the interaction of influence and receptivity, of dominance and submission, and this power can be wielded like a weapon or expressed as a gift.

When negotiated with consent, a power dynamic can be exhilarating, healing, and organizing to a relationship. As an intentional and integrated foundation of a relationship, power exchanges allow one partner to feel their seductive strength while the other feels the sweet release of relinquishing control and decision-making. It allows one person to strategize and lead while the other is taken on a journey. However, when the power dynamic runs the relationship from the shadows, it can inflict harm, stunt personal or relational growth, and create conflict through a desire difference. As an unconscious expression, the power dynamic can emerge in the way we blame a partner instead of taking responsibility for our part, when we withhold parts of ourselves from our partner (either as a protective or punishing gesture), when we dismiss a partner's feelings as less important, or when we take on far too many responsibilities while not having our needs prioritized.

There is so much nuance here that a power dynamic becomes an oftentimes misinterpreted aspect of relationship and therefore a common source of conflict and desire discrepancy. Whether you are consciously engaging it or not, the presence of dominance and submission is pervasive in relationships and must be considered as part of your road map to erotic fulfillment. By inviting the quiet power struggle into the light, you and a partner can learn about who is fulfilling each role, who feels satisfied or frustrated by the role they are in, and what qualities of power turn you on or turn you off. It is not too late to prioritize consent and promote the embodied use of power.

An embodied use of power inspires a deep erotic connection. The partner in the role of dominant can present as a leader for sexual experience, a strong warrior or protector, or a sexual initiator for the partner in the submissive role. When I encourage partners to fully embody the feeling of desire for a partner and physically approach their partner with total-body connectivity and steady acceleration, the partner often responds with disarmed warmth and receptivity.

Likewise, an embodied release into submission can open into a state of deep relaxation and relief. When held with grounded leadership, a receptive partner can learn to let go and turn off the vigilant mind. Also, when the partner in the role of submissive is also in the "bottom" position (meaning the partner receiving the pleasure contact), they can access a euphoric physiological state that the kink or BDSM community refers to as *subspace*. Subspace is accessed when a partner is taken on a sensory journey that may include strong stimulation that activates the sympathetic nervous system for an intense present-moment somatic experience. When engaged with consent, this submissive experience can be personally transformative.

The Erotic Map Guides Your Journey

This chapter has been a step-by-step guide to walking the road of whole-body sex with a partner. Just practicing relationship skills or just investigating your sex life by itself is not enough. By combining the four pillars of embodied relationship as you co-create your erotic map and investigate inevitable desire difference with your partner, you are on the road to a fulfilling relationship and whole-body sexual experience.

10

REFINING THE EROTIC BODY
IN THE WORLD

With your personal awareness now fully awake, thanks to your erotic mapping process and knowledge of the somatic creative process, you can look forward to refining your sexuality and thereby participating in the social change that is so desperately needed in the realm of sexuality at a community level.

Sex and sexual expression are at the root of our most impactful experiences in life. Whether for pleasure or oppression, the experience of sex impacts the core of how we inhabit our bodies. The oppressive side of sex is caused by either an aggressive or silent, avoidance-based mentality—this is what is behind so much unrest and pain in society around our bodies, our sex, and our intimate relationships. An avoidance of sexuality can present itself as misinformation about sexuality, the marginalizing of erotic identities, gender inequality, and barriers to body autonomy (the ability of an individual to make decisions about their own body).

Through recent arousal anatomy and neurobiological research, we are slowly learning to approach sex in more intelligent ways. Activists supporting gender rights, marriage equality, awareness of sexual assault, medical and reproductive body autonomy, and other related causes help to make society aware of the real-life ramifications of body oppression. Unfortunately, we are still far off the mark. Mainstream culture is just beginning to acknowledge the ways societal language and behavior reinforce an oppressive paradigm of sexuality. The public dialogue is clunky as society stumbles through pre-effort expression into a self-reflective place.

In this book, I have hoped to show you that it is possible to cultivate an awake and embodied relationship with your sexuality that honors the personal, spiritual, or cultural values that support body autonomy. By refining

DOI: 10.4324/9780429297236-11

sexuality and arousal, we cultivate more enjoyment and more responsibility over how we express the sexual body. As each of us engages in this process, we grow our collective potential to strike down the systems that reify sexual oppression. In *Decolonizing Sexualities*, researcher and activist Arturo Sanchez Garcia explores the bridging of embodiment with mobilization for collective action. In the Latin American women's movements, personal empowerment allowed for the recognition of the individual as an agent of change. "When a woman recognizes the total experience of her body, acknowledging her own pleasure against the social constructs of desire she can then extend this knowledge and capacity outside of institutionally driven policies to enact fundamental social change" (Bakshi, Jivraj, & Posoccco, 2016, pg. 237). This is the core component of positive social-sexual change for all genders: discovering and self-defining desires while honing a sense of body autonomy in spaces where we feel honored and respected for our authentic embodiment of our somatic self. In a contributing chapter to *Oppression and the Body*, somatic psychotherapist Beit Gorski expresses the desire for all of us to be able tell our stories of body autonomy in every aspect of life. Body autonomy, Gorski says, "is something we can all get behind because, when we release the idea that we control the body, we must then also abandon the rituals of controlling the bodies of others" (Caldwell & Bennett Leighton, 2018, pg. 163).

This book has been a guide to discover that sex is so much more than what society thinks, and fears, it may be. We put so much pressure on genital-focused sex to meet all of our physical, emotional, and intimate needs. When we funnel such important needs through such a small fraction of our expressiveness, we doom ourselves to deep dissatisfaction, resentment, and even destructive or harmful behavior. In these pages, you have been presented with ways to broaden your knowledge and movement repertoire of how you inhabit your body and view the potential of your sexual vitality. The invitation here is to take this information and group of skills into your life to experience sexual vitality in a broader way. Let the wide map of your sexuality take the pressure off the narrow definition of sex to meet your needs and therefore make the sexual experience that you do have more satisfying. When we find pleasure in many places, both sensual and sexual, our sexual shadows are not as scary, and genital-based sex is no longer the basket holding all the eggs—golden eggs are to be found throughout the breadth and depth of your erotic map.

Embodying Your Erotic Revolution and Evolution

After reading this book and engaging in the experientials contained within, you may notice that you are inhabiting your relationship style differently or you may be inhabiting your own expression of sexuality differently. You may find that your public narrative around sex is a little less strained and a little more curious and compassionate. *This is evidence that you are already evolving*. Now is the time to listen to what interests you in your life in order to find your growing edge.

Here is a list of questions to ask yourself as you step into your awakening sexuality:

- Notice the type of activities that you really enjoy. What are the movement qualities you find enjoyable about them? What is your sensory experience of these activities?
- Notice the people that you feel drawn to. What are their personality qualities? What do they represent to you?
- Have your music interests shifted?
- What foods are the most delicious to you now?
- What is happening in your dream life? Make note of the themes, characters, and settings that appear in your dreams.
- Explore the content of your sexual fantasies. Of the fantasy that turns you on the most, evaluate it like a dream (you can use the process found in the section "Erotic Gateways," Chapter 5).
- How are you treating your body? How do you talk to your body? What sensations and emotions arise when relating to your body in sensual or sexual ways? Do you find that your self-talk is more loving and inclusive?
- What aspects of sex that used to be uncomfortable are now neutral or even pleasurable to you?
- How are you responding to the expressions, desires, and fantasies of the important others in your life?

Crafting Your Safe and Inspiring Erotic Spaces

In *Succulent Sexcraft* (2014), Sheri Winston likened the erotic body to an instrument that needs practice and study to learn to play like a master. As we grow and develop brain and body, we dedicate ourselves to the study of history or math, of people or economics, of art and music, or a skilled trade. Rarely do we turn this kind of studied discipline to our sexuality or have the environment to support such a vital study. Now you can create an environment that allows for this kind of study and practice to learn your erotic map. Refining the erotic body is a practice of selecting inspiring and accurate information, engaging with supportive people and communities, and immersing yourself in natural or handcrafted environments that feel safe enough and exciting enough to compel you to continue learning.

What do you know about your preferred and most effective learning style? Do you learn well in a group or are groups too overwhelming or overstimulating for you? Do you enjoy stories or step-by-step instruction (or both)? Do you enjoy reading or listening to information about a topic? I recommend immersive learning tools, whether you are alone or in a group, where you can read, listen, write, and move your body in response to engaging material. Make sure you gather learning tools that are interesting to you and that are within your window of tolerance.

What kind of in-person support feels most interesting and most safe for you right now? Do you want to join a sexuality process group or erotic-themed book club? Can you enlist your partner in co-creative sexy study sessions? Safe community or partner settings can allow for personal exploration and critical thinking that supports holistic growth. If face-to-face interactions feel like a "too soon" suggestion, how about an online study group? I recommend finding a web series or community that is facilitated by a sexuality professional such as a sex therapist, sex counselor, or sex educator. They will be dedicated to creating a safe platform for participants to share and a curriculum for you to follow so that you are not swimming in the uncertain waters of internet chat rooms. Structure and personable support can be a scaffold for you as you integrate your own strength and compassion toward your evolving sexuality.

What environments feel the most conducive and inspiring to your sensual exploration? If your bedroom or another room in the home is the chosen place to explore your sexuality, make sure the space is free of clutter and is aesthetically pleasing to you. You could even create an altar or mandala space nearby with images, objects, smells, and sound-makers that inspire you, turn you on, and help you feel grounded and resilient. You can also place your own erotic map in this space. If the home is not a place to explore, how about the home of a lover or partner, a hotel, a favorite camping or hiking spot, or a dance club? Maybe all of the above! Some environments could be for sensual exploration and some for more explicitly sexual play. Experiment with different spaces and find what works best for you, knowing that this may change over your life span.

In Closing: Your Quest Begins

Remember, your body is magnificent. Your body is both the location of this work and your greatest resource, *not an enemy*, on this path of whole-body sexuality. You have learned how to practice erotic bodyfulness to experience and appreciate your sexual responsiveness. You have created an erotic map to be a guide for deep learning and exploration and you have learned how to combine your erotic map with that of a partner to level up your intimate relationship potential.

While this book is meant to be a guided journey through your somatic landscape to an embodied erotic self, your journey has only just begun. As a quest giver, I charge you with taking the skills detailed in this book and the map that you have developed into your day-to-day life. From this moment on, you have the opportunity to learn, practice, and refine the way that you inhabit your magnificent body. You have everything you need to engage in your life and relationships in a more awake and expressive way, and to ultimately be a part of the larger social change that is already in motion.

My ultimate hope is that through the somatic explorations and creative processes that have been offered here, you have begun to find a home in your erotic body. When you experience your body and your sexuality as a home for your creative potential, you will infuse every space and every relationship with a vibrancy that is contagious. This is just the beginning of the work. From this moment on, you will do the hard work, with discipline, to shine your light into your corner of the world. We all need you to do this. Only then will we collectively appreciate and share in the essential nature of whole-body sexuality.

REFERENCES

Abram, D. (1997). *The spell of the sensuous: Perception and language in a more-than-human world*. Vintage.

Ailey, A. Quote. https://nmaahc.si.edu/blog-post/transforming-dance-around-world.

American Psychiatric Association. (2013). *Diagnostic and statistical manual of mental disorders (DSM-5)*. American Psychiatric Association.

Atkinson, B. (2005). *Emotional intelligence in couples therapy*. Norton Professional Books.

Bainbridge-Cohen, B. www.bodymindcentering.com

Baird, B., & Candelario, R. (2018). *The Routledge companion to butoh performance*. Routledge.

Bakshi, S., Jivraj, S., & Posoccco, S. (2016). *Decolonizing sexualities: Transnational perspectives, critical interventions*. Counterpress.

Basson, R. (2001). Using a different model for female sexual response to address women's problematic low sexual desire. *Sex Marital Therapy*, 27, 395–403.

Basson, R. (2005). Women's sexual dysfunction: Revised and expanded definitions. *Canadian Medical Association Journal*, 172(10), 1327–1333.

Bly, R. (1988). *A little book on the human shadow*. HarperOne.

Braun-Harvey, D., & Vigorito, M. (2015). *Treating out of control sexual behavior: Rethinking sex addiction*. Springer Publishing Company.

Briñol, P., Petty, R.E., & Wagner, R. (2009, August 19). *Body posture effects on self-evaluation: A self-validation approach*. https://doi.org/10.1002/ejsp.607

Caldwell, C. (2016). The moving cycle: A second generation dance/movement therapy form. *American Journal of Dance Therapy*, 38, 245–258.

Caldwell, C. (2018). *Bodyfulness: Somatic practices for presence, empowerment, and waking up in this life*. Shambahla.

Caldwell, C., & Bennett Leighton, L. (2018). *Oppression & the body: Roots, resistance, and resolutions*. North Atlantic Books.

Carrellas, B. (2007). *Urban Tantra: Sacred sex for the 21st century*. Ten Speed Press.

Clark, A. (2010). Empathy: An Integral Model in the Counseling Process. *Journal of Counseling & Development*, 88(Summer), 348–356.

Constantides, D. (2019). *Sex therapy with erotically marginalized clients*. Routledge.

Cornell, A. (1996). *The power of focusing: A practical guide to emotional self-healing*. New Harbinger Publications.

Cozolino, L. (2006). *The neuroscience of human relationships: Attachment and the developing social brain*. W. W. Norton & Company, Inc.

Cozolino, L. (2017). *The neuroscience of psychotherapy: Healing the social brain*. W. W. Norton & Company, Inc.

Csikszentmihalyi, M. (2014). *Flow, the secret to happiness*. TED Talk.

Daley, E. (2020). *Embodied consent: A somatic approach to sexual wellness*. Unpublished masters thesis.

Damasio, A. (1994). *Descartes error: Emotion, reason, and the human brain*. Penguin Books.

Desikachar, T.K.V. (1995). *The heart of yoga: Developing a personal practice*. Inner Traditions.

Desmond, J. (2001). *Dancing desires: Choreographing sexualities on and off stage*. University of Wisconsin Press.

Easton, D. & Hardy, J. (2017). *The ethical slut: A practical guide to polyamory, open relationships, and other freedoms in sex and love*. Ten Speed Press.

Ekman, P. (2003). *Unmasking the face: A guide to recognizing emotions from facial expressions*. Malor Books.

Ellison, C.R. (2006). *Women's sexualities: Generations of women share intimate secrets of sexual self-acceptance*. Read File Publishing Company.

Frank, R. (2001). *Body of awareness: A Somatic and developmental approach to psychotherapy*. Gestalt Press.

Fredrickson, B. (2013). Positive emotions broaden and build. *Advances in Experimental Social Psychology*, 47, Elsevier Inc. ISSN 0065–2601.

Gibson, R. (2008). *My body my earth: The practice of somatic archaeology*. iUniverse.

Gladwell, M. (2005). *Blink: The power of thinking without thinking*. Back Bay Books.

Hackney, P. (2002). *Making connections: Total body integration through Bartenieff fundamentals*. Routledge.

Haines, S. (2007). *Healing sex: A mind-body approach to healing sexual trauma*. Cleis Press.

Haradon, G., Bascom, B., Dragomir, C., & Scripcaru, V. (1994). Sensory functions of institutionalized Romanian infants: A pilot study. *Occupational Therapy International*, 1(4), 250–260.

Johnson, S. (2013). *Love sense: The revolutionary new science of romantic relationships*. Little, Brown Spark.

Jung, C. (1952). *The integration of personality*. Routledge & Kegan Paul.

Keleman, S. (1985). *Emotional anatomy: The structure of experience*. Center Press.

Kestenberg-Amighi, J., Loman, S., & Sossin, K.M. (2018). *The meaning of movement: Embodied development, clinical, and cultural perspectives of the Kestenberg Movement Profile*. Routledge.

Kim, T.I., Shin, Y.H., & White-Traut, R. (2003). Multisensory intervention improves physical growth and illness rates in Korean orphaned newborn infants. *Research in Nursing Health*, 26: 424–433.

Klein, M. (2012). *Sexual intelligence: What we really want from sex and how to get it*. HarperOne.

Kleinman, S. (1983). *Sexuality and the dance*. National Dance Association of the American Alliance for Health, Physical Education, Recreation, and Dance, Reston, VA.

Kleinplatz, P. (2012). *New directions in sex therapy: Innovations and alternatives, 2nd Edition*. Brunner-Routledge.

Kurtz, R. (1990). *Body-centered psychotherapy: The Hakomi method*. LifeRhythm.

Laban, R. von (1974). *The language of movement: A guidebook to choreutics*. Plays, Inc.

Lorde, A. (1978). *Uses of the erotic: The erotic as power*. Out & Out Books.

Martin, B. www.bettymartin.org

Masters, W.H., & Johnson, V.E. (1966). *Human sexual response*. Toronto and New York: Bantam Books.

Morin, J. (1996). *The erotic mind: Unlocking the inner sources of passion and fulfillment*. Harper Perennial.

Nagoski, E. (2015). *Come as you are: The Surprising new science that will transform your sex life*. Simon & Schuster.

O'Donahue, J. (1998). *Anam cara: A book of celtic wisdom*. Harper Collins.

Ogden, G. (2015). *Extraordinary sex therapy: Creative approaches for clinicians*. Routledge.

Pallaro, P. (1999). *Authentic Movement: Essays by Mary Starks Whitehouse, Janet Adler and Joan Chodorow*. Jessica Kingsly Publishers.

Patterson, A. (2019). *The secret to female vitality*. Ebook.

Pelmas, C. (2017). *Trauma: A practical guide to working with body and soul (Somatic Sex Educator's Handbook Book 1)*. CreateSpace Independent Publishing Platform.

Pinkola Estes, C. (1996). *Women who run with the wolves: Myths and stories of the wild woman archetype*. Ballantine Books.

Pitagora, D. (2017). No pain, no gain?: Therapeutic and relational benefits of subspace in BDSM contexts. *Journal of Positive Sexuality*, 3(3), 44–54, Widener University.

Porges, S. (2011). *The polyvagal theory: Neurophysiological foundations of emotions, attachment, communication, and self-regulation*. W. W. Norton & Company.

Reich, W. (1986). *Selected writings: An introduction to orgonomy*. Farrar, Straus and Giroux.

Resnick, S. (2018). *Body-to-body intimacy: Transformation through love, sex, and neurobiology*. Routledge.

Roth, G. (1998). *Maps to ecstasy: The healing power of movement*. New World Library.

Rothschild, B. (2000). *The body remembers: The psychophysiology of trauma and trauma treatment*. W. W. Norton & Co.

Schwartz, A. Quote. drarielleschwartz.com/somatic-therapy-in-trauma-treatment-dr-arielle-schwartz

Seoane, K. (2016). Parenting the self with self-applied touch: A dance/movement therapy approach to self-regulation. *American Journal of Dance Therapy*, 38, 21–40.

Siegel, D. (2010). *Mindsight: The new science of personal transformation*. Bantam.

Tantia, J.F. (2012). Authentic movement and the autonomic nervous system: A preliminary investigation. *American Journal of Dance Therapy*, 34(1), 53–73.

Tatkin, S. (2012). *Wired for love: How understanding your partners brain and attachment style can help you defuse conflict and build a secure relationship*. New Harbinger Publications.

Treleaven, D.A. (2018). *Trauma-sensitive mindfulness: Practices for safe and transformative healing*. W. W. Norton & Co.

Turner, T. (2017). *Belonging: Remembering ourselves home*. Her Own Room Press.

Van der Kolk, B. (1989). *The compulsion to repeat the trauma: Re-enactment, revictimization, and masochism*. Psychiatric Clinics of North America, Vol. 12:2, pgs. 389-411.

van der Kolk, B. (2015). *The body keeps the score: Brain, mind, and body in the healing of trauma*. Penguin Books.

Veaux, F., & Rickert, E. (2014). *More than two: A practical guide to polyamory*. Thorntree Press.

Wade, J. (2004). *Transcendent sex: When lovemaking opens the veil*. Gallery Books.

Weaver, L. (2018). *Luminous: Poems and inquiry for the soul's journey*. Laura Weaver.

Weiner, L., & Avery-Clark, C. (2017). *Sensate focus in sex therapy: The illustrated manual.* Routledge.

Weiss, G. (1998). *Body images: Embodiment as intercorporeality.* Routledge.

Whipple, B., & Brash-McGreer, K. (1997). Management of female sexual dysfunction. In M.L. Sipski & C. Alexander (Eds.), *Sexual function in people with disability and chronic illness: A health professional's guide* (pp. 511–536). Gaithersburg, MD: Aspen Publishers.

Winks, C., & Seamans, K. (2002). *Good vibrations guide to sex: The most complete sex manual ever written.* Cleis Press.

Winston, S. (2010). *Women's anatomy of arousal: Secret maps to buried pleasure.* Mango Garden Press.

Winston, S. (2014). *Succulent sexcraft: Your hands-on guide to erotic play and practice.* Mango Garden Press.

Zolbrod, A. (2009). *SexSmart: How your childhood shaped your sexual life and what to do about it.* iUniverse.

Zweig, C., & Abrams, J. (1991). *Meeting the shadow: The hidden power of the dark side of human nature.* TarcherPerigree.

INDEX

Note: Page numbers in *italics* indicate a figure on the corresponding page.

5Rhythms dance 16–17, 26, 130

Abram, David 26, 104
Ailey, Alvin 66
animated flow 45
archetypes 159–160
arousal 87–90, 97–101, 120
arousal anatomy 2–3
arousal non-concordance 80, 84, 121
asexual 3, 79
authentic movement 42–43, 67, 116
automated sexual self 157
Avery-Clark, Constance 36

Bainbridge-Cohen, Bonnie 39
Bartenieff Fundamentals (Hackney) 48
Bartenieff, Irmgard 11, 121
Basson, Rosemary 79
Beauty and the Beast 160
belly brain 61
Belonging (Turner) 41
bipolar shape flow 49–50
Blink: The Power of Thinking Without Thinking (Gladwell) 29
body armor 9, 19, 54, 68, 101, 107–108, 120, 142; arousal and 158; breathing and 59; in character structure 40; coping strategies as 153; as defense mechanisms 8, 55, 67; emotions and 84;

in nonconsensual sex 2; in relational space 76
Body as Shadow, The (Conger) 20
body autonomy 2, 37–38, 108, 179–180
bodyfulness 53, 55, 77
body-half connection 124
body language 27–28
body rhythms 45–46
Body-to-Body Intimacy (Resnick) 36, 89
bound tension-flow 45
Braun-Harvey, Douglas 155
breath support 122–123

Caldwell, Christine 29, 41–42, 53; *see also* Moving Cycle model
character structure 40
circular model of sexual response 79, 85
Come as You Are (Nagoski) 37
committed relationships 30–31
community, role of embodied sexuality in 113–114
consensual sex 2
consent 133; embodied 100–101; informed 100–101
core/distal connectivity 124
core erotic theme 158
Cosmopolitan 7
Cozolino, Louis 6
cross-lateral connection 124
Csikszentmihalyi, Mihaly 55

cultural oppression of body 106–107
culture 105, 111–112, 179

D'Abate, Leah 62
dance/movement therapy (DMT) 1, 42, 65, 67, 71, 116, 118, 133
Dancing Desires (Desmond) 117
Decolonizing Sexualities (Bakshi, Jivraj, and Posoccco) 108, 180
defense mechanisms 8
desire for intimacy 121
divided sexual self 8–10
Doyle, Arthur Conan 21
dynamic alignment 126–128
dysregulated reactions 153–154

efforts 49
Ekman, Paul 21
Ellison, Carol Rinkleib 75
embeddedness 103–106
embodied consent 100–101
embodied erotic self 1, 182
embodied expressiveness 14
embodied intimacy, pillars of: balance between safety and novelty 168–169; communication and expressiveness 165–167; self-awareness 163–165; sexual intelligence 167–168
embodied movement 44
embodied sex 34
embodied sexuality 14, 33, 113–114, 133, 167, 175–176
embodied sexual self 30, 50
embodied touch 132–134
embodiment 13, 29, 36, 42, 46, 103, 107–108, 119; as a diverse experience 108; by whiteness 107
environmental anchor 58
erotic 116; definition 56–57; path to savoring 72–73
erotic awareness 51
erotic body 1, 11, 13, 21, 31–32, 45, 52, 75, 77–78, 82, 106–107, 116–117, 121, 158, 181, 183
erotic bodyfulness 2, 12–13, 57–58, 72, 100–101, 117; activation of trauma and 54–56; experience of sexual allyship 112–113; experience of sexual ecology 110–111; in nonsexual realm 71–72
erotic bodyfulness sequence: breathing with intention 59–60; identifying anchor 58–59; inviting movement impulses 65–68; mind's awareness of

body 60–62; movement impulses 64–65; oscillating attention 62–63; pleasure movement and yield response 68–69; points of sensation 63–64
erotic energy 14, 71, 141
erotic intelligence 26
eroticism 8, 14–15, 38, 52, 83, 139, 143, 155–158, 169; embodied 11; front and back body connection 130; intelligent 97; mindful 36; obstacle aspect of 22
erotic map 2, 14–15, 78, 139–140, *142*, 179; application of 161; autopilot movement on *156*; combining 163, 169–175, *170*; conflict between 176–178; core erotic self on 158; dysregulated movement pattern of *154*; for non-monogamy and polyamory 175; *see also* erotic mapping process, realms of
erotic mapping process, realms of: core erotic theme 158–161; dysregulated reactions 153–154; eroticism 155–157; finding challenges 147–148; gateways 150–151; interest and obstacle 145–147; mastery and easeful effort 141–145; reactive habitual movement patterns 153–154; resilience 151–153, *152*; resource 144–145; shadows 148–150
erotic revolution and evolution 180–181
erotic self 1, 5, 8, 14–15, 26, 106, 158
erotic spaces 181–182
erotoceptive senses 36

familial and social impact on sexuality 36–37
fight-flight-freeze response 100
fixation 62
focus during sex 35–36
Footloose 118
Frank, Ruella 30
Freehill, Maureen Momo 115–116
free tension-flow 45
friendships 39
full-bodied sexuality 119
full-effort erotic expressiveness 121–122, 138; breath support 122–123; dynamic alignment 126–128; sequenced movement 124–126; spatial intent 128–130

Garcia, Arturo Sanchez 180
gateways 150–151
gender embodiment 13, 36
Good Vibrations Guide to Sex, The (Winks and Semans) 79, 103
Gorski, Beit 180

habitual relational patterns 30
Haines, Staci 19
head-tail connectivity 124
Heart of Yoga, The (Desikachar) 59
holistic sexual self 10
human intersubjectivity 104

informed consent 100–101
interpersonal empathy 105
intimacy 1–2, 9, 13, 26, 34, 48–49,
    54, 58, 79–80, 86, 89, 103, 117, 146,
    162; desire for 121; embodied intimacy
    163–169; joyful 2; over efficiency
    169

joyful intimacy 2; *see also* intimacy
jumping rhythm 47–48, 171
Jung, Carl 104

Kennedy, Ryan 44
Kestenberg Movement Profile (KMP)
    44–45
kinesphere 44, 78, 129
Klein, Marty 35
Kleinplatz, Peggy 23, 34
Kolk, Bessel van der 7

Laban, Rudolf 21, 77
Little Book on the Human Shadow, A
    (Bly) 18
lived experience of being 2
Lorde, Audre 14

Martin, Betty 133
Michaels, Melissa 16–17, 26, 130
mindful eroticism 36
mindfulness practices 1, 36, 52–53,
    55, 58
mirror neurons 104–105
mistrust of body 8
moment-to-moment practice of
    embodied movement 42–44
moment-to-moment sexual self 32, 34
*More Than Two: A Practical Guide to
    Polyamory* (Veaux and Rickert) 129
Morin, Jack 22, 158
mother-tongue language of body 31–32,
    42, 56–58
Moving Cycle model 41–42; action phase
    42; appreciation phase 42; awareness
    phase 41; owning
    phase 42
Mozart in the Jungle (DeSousa) 116

Nagoski, Emily 23, 54, 80
naval radiation, pathway of 124
neutral flow 45
New Directions in Sex Therapy
    (Kleinplatz) 34, 105
nonconsensual sex 22
nonlinear model of sexual response 79

obstacles: in eroticism 22; of non-erotic
    kind 23–24
Oppression and the Body (Bennett
    Leighton) 107, 180
organicity 151
out of control sexual behavior (OCSB) 156

Parish, Ramon 73
Patterson, Alicia 9
Paxton, Steven 126
Pelmas, Christiane 15
Perel, Esther 119
performance-based sex 34
Peter Pan 160
physiological distress 9
pleasure 2, 4–8, 13, 22, 33–34, 39–41, 43,
    51–52, 54–58, 68–69, 81–85; body
    movement and 31, 71; emotional
    5–7; physical 5; self-pleasure 133,
    160, 167; sexuality as 4; *see also*
    sensations
polyvagal theory 54
Porges, Stephen 7, 54
Power of Focusing, The (Cornell) 41
pre-efforts 49, 107, 118–119
prefrontal cortex 19, 76
Princess Bride, The 97
psychological kinesphere 129

*Queering/Querying the Body: Sensation
    and Curiosity in Disrupting Body Norms*
    (Johnson) 105

reactive habitual movement patterns
    153–154
Reich, Wilhelm 40
relational space/field 13, 20, 76
resilience 151–153
resilient sexual self 10–11
Resnick, Stella 61
rhythmic movement strategies 45–46
romantic relationships 8, 39
Roth, Gabrielle 16
Rothschild, Babette 58
running/drifting 46

satisfaction cycle 39–40
Savasana 130
Scarlet Letter, The (Hawthorne) 106
School of Body-Mind Centering 39
self-applied touch 133–134
Sensate Focus in Sex Therapy (Weiner and Avery-Clark) 36, 133
sensations 38, 41–42, 56–57, 63–64, 95, 117; *see also* pleasure
Sensuality and the Dance (Ossosky) 117
Seoane, Kendra 133
sequenced movement 124–126
sex-as-performance model 75
sex education 8
sex-negative experiences 119
sex therapy 1; *see also* somatic sex therapy
sexual accelerators and brakes 23–24
sexual allyship 112–113
sexual arousal 22, 54–55, 82, 97–101, 167
sexual consent 2
sexual diversity 36
sexual ecology 103, 106–111
sexual energy 11, 101
sexual environment 106, 108, 140
Sexual Excitation System (SES) 24, 55, 136
sexual fantasies 22–23
Sexual Inhibition System (SIS) 24, 54, 136
sexuality 1–5, 9, 11, 13, 15, 17, 19, 32, 37–38, 76–77, 112, 181; dynamic alignment in 126; experience and expression of 5; familial and social impact on 36–37; presentation of 7; social-sexual environment and 108–111; societal map of 14
sexuality information 13
sexuality shadow 20–21
sexual pre-efforts 49
sexual response cycle 78–80; arousal non-concordance 80; map 101–102; *see also* whole-body sexual response cycle
sexual self 5, 7–9, 11, 13, 75, 121
sexual shame 2, 6
sexual wellness 77–78
shadow movements 20–21, 77, 172
shadows 17, 19–21, 24–25, 148–150
shaming paradigm of sexuality 118
shape flow 49–50
Singer-Kaplan, Helen 79
skin-to-skin contact 132
Skyler, Jenni 34
small dance 126

snapping/biting 47
social ecology *109*
social engagement system (SES) 55, 134
social inhibition system (SIS) 8
social nervous system 6
social-sexual environment 108–111
sociocultural environment 2
solo sex (masturbation) 9, 23, 73, 117–118, 133, 160, 162
somatic anchor 58
somatic architecture 10, 28, 58
somatic armor 9, 24, 40, 55
somatic awareness 41–42, 46, 50, 151
somatic-based sexuality 17; *see also* sexuality
somatic (body-based) psychotherapy 1
Somatic-Concentric Sex Therapy (S-CST) 1–3, 11, *12*
somatic creative process 38–41
somatic map 44–45, 52
somatic self 1–2, 38, 43, 49, 73
somatic sex therapy 31–33
somatic sexual self 15, 103
somatophobia 29
somatosensory experience of body 11–12
somatosensory language 28, 31–32
spatial intent 128–130
Spell of the Sensuous (Abram) 103–104
spurting/ramming rhythm 47
starting/stopping 47
strain/release 47
subjective empathy 105
Succulent Sexcraft (Winston) 181
sucking rhythm 46
surging/birthing 47, 144
swaying rhythm 46

talk therapy 1
Temple of Apollo 53
tension-flow attributes 48
tension-flow rhythms: fighting 47; indulging 46–47
total body connectivity 122, 124, 133, 138, 143, 161, 163, 178
touch-based mindfulness practice 36
touching: between partners 135; consent and 133; embodied touch 132–138; in erotic bodyfulness practice 136–137; self-applied touch 133–134; skin-to-skin contact 132
transition between movements and rhythms 47–48
Treleaven, David A. 55

triphasic model 79
twisting rhythm 46

unipolar shape flow 50
upper-lower connection 124

Wakefield, Chelsea 159
Weiner, Linda 36
Weiss, Gail 103
"Wheel of Consent" 133
Whitehouse, Mary Starks 28, 42
whole-body sexuality 103, 162, 182–183
whole-body sexual response cycle 80–82,
    81; arousal 87–90, 97–100; concentric

model of arousal 98; embedded center
and surrounding context 94–96; erotic
gateways 82–85; flow space 90–91;
integration 93–94; peak moments
91–93; sexual desire 85–87; transitions
96; *see also* sexual response cycle
whole-person sexual responsiveness 2
wild self 25–26
Winston, Sheri 75
Women's Sexualities (Ellison) 34
Women Who Run With the Wolves
    (Pinkola Estes) 159

Zolbrod, Aline 37

9780367276720